CW01664904

Soul Journeys

An Exploration in Multi-Dimensional Consciousness

Kimberley Lovell

Soul Journeys. An Exploration in Multi-Dimensional Consciousness.

Copyright © 2022 Kimberley Lovell.

All rights reserved. This book or any portion thereof may not be reproduced or used in any manner whatsoever without the express written permission of the publisher except for the use of brief quotations in a book review.

ISBN: 978-1-7397909-1-2

Authors Website: www.KimberleyLovell.co.uk Sign up here to access Book Bonuses

YouTube Channel: Kimberley Lovell

Soulutions Publishing, Rainbow Lodge, Bournemouth, Dorset BH10 6BN England

Front & Back Book Cover: *Original Image Credit: NASA, ESA, and A. Nota (STScI/ESA)*, cropping/positioning and slight re-colouring by Kimberley Lovell

Book Meditation Bonuses: https://bit.ly/SJ1BookBonus

Contents

Acknowledgements

I would like to acknowledge and thank all those who have guided, inspired, empowered, and supported me over many years to be all who I am and who I continue to become. My teachers, coaches, mentors, peers, my beloved spirit guides, star beings, ascended masters, my beautiful goddess sisters, friends and soul family, my clients, and students for whom it has been my greatest joy and privilege to witness the amazing transformations that have unfolded and continue to unfold in their lives.

A special thanks for the beautiful souls who were kind enough to allow me to share their magical sessions with you. You know who you are.

My amazing team of beta readers who volunteered to read my draft manuscript. Thank you for your invaluable feedback.

My beloved partner for his constant love, support, and encouragement in all I do.

You my beloved readers who without knowing have called this book into being. My love and gratitude to you all.

This book is dedicated to
Mother/Father God/Goddess, Creator of All That Is

To Mother Earth, and All within the Nature
and Animal Kingdom

To all beings on this universal
and cosmic journey of Ascension.

With love, honour, and gratitude
for the gift that you be.

Foreword

We are living through some of the most troubling times of our lives and of the planet. Now, more than ever, the future of humanity and the Earth depends on a critical mass of people connecting with their purpose, with who and what they really are, and with the great spiritual truths that underlie everything about why we're here.

Ever more people are turning to the esoteric and mystical truths that are the foundation of true religion, spirituality, humanity, and nature, and there are more and more powerful routes we can take to travel inwards. One of those is the connections we may make with angels, star beings, and our own past lives.

One of the saving graces for humanity right now is the wealth of practitioners and resources available for each of us to choose the path or paths that will take us up the mountain of self-knowledge. Here is one of those.

My own journey has been broad, passing through several religions (briefly or for a longer while), various philosophies and practices, and into contact with innumerable practitioners. Connecting with my personal guardian angel several years ago, and developing my relationship with him – something that had occurred over several lifetimes – has been one of my single greatest learnings and insights.

There is so much we can know, that we can keep on exploring our entire lives. Some encounters will be more meaningful than others, but being open to looking – seeking – is a requirement of living.

Kimberley is a precious soul, with the deepest warmth and caring, who it's been my pleasure to know for a few years now. I'm excited she's sharing these fascinating transcripts and providing another window into the kinds of journeys we can embark on.

Sue Fitzmaurice
Author, Editor, Publisher

Preface

I have spent over 37 years working with spirit, as a medium, channel, healer, coach, business mentor, spiritual teacher and trainer in many holistic healing modalities, empowering my clients and students through utilising the power of the subconscious, superconscious mind, hypnosis, and energy healing empowering them to connect more fully with their unconscious, their higher self, spirit guides and most importantly their intuition. I feel truly honoured to be able to facilitate this work and to support my clients in connecting with their guides and multi-dimensional aspects, to gain valuable insight, wisdom, healing, and resources and to transform the unconscious limiting beliefs, emotions, and behaviours, integrating mind, body, spirit, and emotions, and creating a rich, soulful, and fulfilling, life and business. This is part of our soul's journey and the process of ascension.

I had trained in counselling, transpersonal hypnotherapy, and numerous other healing modalities and was teaching a variety of personal and spiritual development workshops, and holistic training courses before setting up my own transpersonal hypnotherapy training school. I have a wonderful spirit team who work with me, consisting of many ascended masters, archangels, and galactic star-beings who are a part of the white brotherhood/ sisterhood. I have myself been channelling these beings on and off over the years so I had always known I would write a book, but *this* was not the book that I intended to write.

I had been guided to take my past life regression module from my hypnotherapy training, update it and teach it online. I decided that I would record several hypnotherapy sessions online so that I would have a substantial training vault of hypnotherapy sessions for my students to supplement the live online training. Having recorded and transcribed over 30 hours of hypnotherapy sessions, I was told by Spirit, that not only were these sessions to form part of the training, but that Spirit also desired for the information to be shared more widely in a book format to support humanity in understanding how hypnosis can support the multi-dimensional soul's journey and the ascension process.

Some of these sessions were 60 minutes, some were 90 minutes or longer. Some were simple past life regression, others spent more time in the life between lives, galactic lives, or channelling various galactic star beings. All of these sessions were recorded for this purpose and all participants have agreed for the material to be used. All but one of the sessions took place online and were recorded in 2020 and transcribed. For the purposes of privacy, I have changed client names and edited out any personal identifying information.

I have struggled to name each chapter as there was so much within each session, with client's dipping in and out of past life, life between life, future life, healing activations, light language, contact with galactic beings, and channelling. Each session is rather like a spiritual mystery tour, rich in insight, wisdom and carries keys and codes for our soul's journey. Each person's experience of trance and regression is different, sometimes it flows, sometimes it can feel a little disjointed and whilst we're working with the unconscious mind, the conscious mind is always in the background to a greater or lesser degree. In trance, the client's experience and dialogue can switch between first-person and third person with the level of trance they're experiencing and depending on whether they are seeing, hearing, or feeling at the time. Sometimes the client flows, sometimes I'm asking a lot of questions to orientate the client and keep them moving forward. When in hypnosis, our speech and grammatical sentence structure can be less coherent with stopping and starting of sentences. I have tried to leave as much of the natural language as possible and have restructured some of the sentences to make them easier for reading and understanding.

Humanity is on the brink of a quantum leap in consciousness. In this time of ascension that is prophesied and known as the Golden Age, it is our task individually and collectively to awaken to our Soul origins, our multi-dimensionality, our soul's potential, to create a more conscious, illuminated, and enlightened world, where we co-create with Source, with the Earth, all of nature and with one another. Our invitation stands as it always has to live our heaven on earth. The future of humanity and of our beloved blue planet Earth depends on us. We are the ones.

This book contains many keys and codes that will unlock your own soul's journey for it is energetically encoded with the sacred crystalline Christos Sophia energies of New Earth, the Heaven on Earth that we are collectively co-creating. It is my hope that you will find that the material shared within this book will illuminate, enlighten, and inspire you to awaken, connect and align more fully with your Soul's journey, to explore your multi-dimensionality and to start or continue your own personal and spiritual ascension journey of self-mastery and sovereignty.

May this journey and co-creation of awakening souls bring you much love, light, joy, peace, and fulfilment.

With love and blessings from my heart to yours

Kimberley

Interested to discover more about your own soul's journey? Further information and resources regarding 1:1 sessions, quantum hypnotherapy training, hypnotic meditations, soul journey ascension programme can be found on my website. www.KimberleyLovell.co.uk

Oak Tree

I may look dead
But fear not
I am alive and well
For it is in the darkness of winter
That I release and renew
That I fortify
Embracing the quiet and the solitude
As I simply let go
And go within
For hidden deep within
At the core of my being
Is the light
The seed
The blueprint
For my renewal and resurrection
For all of life dies
Only to be reborn
I like you am
An Infinite Being
Of Light
We are infinite love
For all of life is eternal.
In the darkness and winter of life
Send your roots down even deeper
Connecting with the core of the Earth
For the earth is our Mother
Feel into your connection
With all of life
All of nature

Send your light down
Notice how our roots and branches are connected
To each other
Send your light up
Like open arms outstretched
Through each and every branch
See how our branches almost touch
Allow the soul light to flow
Through the network of roots and branches
Beneath the crystalline grids of Mother Earth
As our hearts and souls unite
For our branches
Reach to the stars in heaven
Reminding us of our true nature
Our true home
Our roots connecting with these ancient lands
And with our ancestors in whose footsteps, we tread
As we remember to walk
In unity and love
As the beings of light we are
Brothers and Sisters
One Family
United we Stand Tall
Together
A circle of Love
Embracing all of life

© Kimberley Lovell 2021
Channelled from the Young Oak Tree in my garden, which was Divinely Gifted and Seeded by The Winged Ones (Bird Tribe)

Introduction to Past Life Regression Theories

This book will reach both newcomers and those who are more familiar with this work. Before I share these sessions with you. I thought it might be helpful for some of you to understand a little more about this work.

Time: Past, Present, Future Lives, Parallel Lives

Time is not linear, it is simultaneous. Everything including the past and the future is happening at the same time. Time is a manufactured 3D construct. In our 3D reality time is linear, but in higher dimensions, time doesn't exist. If we extend this thinking, we are multi-dimensional beings, living and existing throughout time and space in many dimensions in one form or another. Past lives, future lives, life between lives, galactic lives then are actually parallel lives.

Reincarnation and Past Lives

For those who accept the idea that we live many lives through reincarnation, one past-life theory is that during regression the consciousness goes back into a past life incarnation.

DNA/Genetic/Ancestral Memory

Another theory is that we enter into the memory of an ancestor, such as our great-grandparents, great grandparents, or so on. The mapping of the human genome has uncovered the inclusion of long strings of so-called junk DNA. These undecipherable strands of DNA might play a role in racial or ancestral memories. This theory is based on the concept that the neo-cortex inherits memories through the genes or held within the morphogenetic field. Irresistible urges such as the instinct to procreate and nurture children are said to be genetic imprints on the psyche. Therefore, racial, or ancestral memories, fears, phobias, trauma, maybe soft coded in specific genes or held within the morphogenetic field.

Examples of such inherited memories abound in nature. For example, a sheepdog separated from any dogs of his breed at birth will still demonstrate a natural skill for herding. Sheepdog owners report their dogs will attempt to herd any groups they come across from human children to sheep. Scientists refer to this as a genetic memory inherited from the parents. This theory is based upon the concept that humans inherit memories their ancestors accumulate until the age they bear their first child. This means that if your great, great, great grandmother had her first child at the age of 18 her life experience only until age 18 would be stored in her descendants' memories.

Mediumship

Others assert that the experiences that become known during past life regression are a form of mediumship; or channelling a personality from beyond death. This theory suggests that past lives are the memories of someone else who once lived. The hypnotic trance state then opens lines of communication with spirits living in another state or dimension.

Fantasy

Another theory suggests that all so-called past life memories are constructs of the subconscious or unconscious mind. The subconscious feels they are 'real' the same way dreams are real.

False Memory

Other researchers say that because suggestion is part of hypnosis, subjects under past life hypnosis develop past life images and material because of implied or explicit suggestions by the therapist that the subject examines his/her previous lives.

Imprinting

During past life regression sessions, sometimes clients are shown famous historical figures lives Sometimes the client is sure they are the person, and other times they can feel like they're making it up. Yet the client is not making it up and doesn't know the difference between a real past life or an imprint, because both are experienced in the same way. i.e., the client experiences them in the same way they would a real past life. Hearing, seeing, or sensing, depending on their individual gifts and abilities.

I have experienced this personally within a hypnosis session many years ago, whereas a client in a hypnosis session that was not a past life regression, a past life spontaneously surfaced, and I experienced myself as Mary and I was sobbing and 'wailing for my lord who is on the cross.' All the while, whilst still sobbing, I remember thinking, Kim you weren't Mother Mary or Mary

Magdalene. Years later whilst on a theta healing instructor training, I spontaneously, experienced myself as Jesus on the cross. Whilst I do feel close to Jesus/Yeshua, Mother Mary, and Mary Magdalene, and feel that I was present in those times, and often channel them, I know that I wasn't them. I now know them to be part of my spirit team, they are wonderful guides on the inner planes. I believe my experience was either imprinting from my higher Self, mediumship, or connection with the Akashic Records. In both of those sessions, my experience was about suffering, sacrifice loss, and the wounded healer's journey of ascension as we transmute the pain, heal our hearts, and transform our consciousness. I have also had many clients who experienced themselves as famous historical figures and obviously we can't all be the same person. There are a couple of sessions in the book where the client has a similar experience relating to other historical figures.

Conclusion

The fact is that whether past lives can ever be proven or not these methods have proven to work in therapy. Hypnotic regression allows the individual to temporarily dissociate from their present problematic reality and express feelings and thoughts they fear. They might be past lives, images from the subconscious, imprints, or hallucinations but they are therapeutic and often correlate to the client's present life issues. Resolution of the past life/parallel life gift them great insight, wisdom, resources, healing setting them free to be more of who they truly are in this life.

Six Criteria for Determining Validity of a Past Life Experience

True past life experiences are accompanied by intense emotions that seem to come from nowhere. This could be experienced as:

- A strong sense of déjà vu regarding a place.
- Intense familiarity when meeting someone for the first time.
- An intensely emotional and/or kinetic feeling during hypnotic trance.
- The emergence of previously unknown (unstudied) talents.
- Knowledge of unknowable historical details.
- Discovering that others share your memories.

Possible alternative explanations for these experiences are:

Metaphors

The past life images and experiences are metaphors for the individual's current life challenges. For example, a woman who feels used and cheated by everyone may discover a past life as a frail young slave woman who never protested the injustice she suffered.

Collective Unconscious (Akashic Record)

That the individual has tapped into the Akashic Record (sometimes called the Collective Unconscious.) Both names refer to records that contain all knowledge of human experience and the history of the cosmos. These records are metaphorically described as a library, a universal computer, or the Mind of God.

Attachments & Spirit Release

Some attribute the information accessed in past life hypnosis to the invasion, possession, or influence of the individual by entities/spirits. Possession is when an individual is taken over by an entity/spirit. This is attributed to the fact that on occasion victims of so-called possession attain access to hidden knowledge, foreign languages, and drastic changes in voice or even appearance. Throughout history diseases that were beyond understanding such as Epilepsy were attributed to the presence of a vengeful spirit or in the body of the patient.

Past Life/Parallel Life Integration

The past life integration technique is a transformative process that reconnects the individual to his or her immortal nature. By regaining insight and awareness of past lives and healing any past life trauma we integrate the past life/parallel life into our consciousness. This means that any power or creativity developed by our past life or parallel personalities may be channelled into our current day-to-day reality. Conscious awareness of our past lives provides us with an ongoing connection to our immortal nature. The benefits of past life integration transcend our day-to-day problems and challenges. It's possible to carry an awareness of our past lives into future lives as well. When we can accomplish this, we become fearless. When we are living proof that death is nothing but a transition from one experience, one body, to the next we develop profound compassion for all. This comes from a place of ease and acceptance once we understand that we ourselves have in fact lived lives as many different kinds of people. As the old nursery rhyme goes *Tinker, Tailor, Soldier, Sailor, Rich Man, Poor Man, Beggar Man, Thief.*

The African Warrior

This client was a young lady of African descent. She was recommended to me by another client and was keen to explore past life regression for the first time. She's an actor, open to, but not really well-versed in spirituality and the soul's journey. She was keen to explore past life regression and she wanted to discover more about her Soul purpose and if she was on the right track with her career.

TP: I'm in a forest; it's a bit fluffy really, but there's a settlement and like mud huts almost.

KL: What type of trees are there?

TP: Short ones; quite sandy actually. Quite sandy and muddy.

KL: So just take a moment to look down at your feet and see what you're wearing?

TP: I'm barefoot

KL: As you look up at your body, do you have any clothes?

TP: Something short.

KL: Are you male or female?

TP: I'm Female.

KL: What kind of age are you? How does your body feel?

TP: I'd say quite young; somewhere between mid-teens to early twenties.

KL: Okay, and what's your name?

TP: I'm not sure.

KL: Just allow yourself to be in this space, in the forest, feeling your feet on the earth. Is there anyone else around?

TP: Yeah, families; everyone in the community.

KL: Is there anyone there that you recognise? Is your family there?

TP: I don't think I can see my specific family, but I do know all the people there.

KL: What do they call you? (silence) It doesn't matter; you can allow a name to come to you later. Tell me more about the settlement, where is it?

TP: Somewhere hot? Feels like either somewhere in Africa or America.

KL: What are people doing?

TP: There are people talking, making stuff, playing, laughing, looking after the family.

KL: I wonder where your family is?

TP: They're inside.

KL: How many people are there in your family? Do you have siblings?

TP: Two brothers—one older; one younger.

KL: What are their names?

TP: I'm not sure yet.

KL: Okay. Let's move forward. Let's just condense time; we can easily do that. As we move forward in time, let's move forward to the next significant time. Tell me what happens.

TP: How far are we moving forward?

KL: I don't know. I wonder. You can move forward in this lifetime, or you may find yourself going somewhere else. (silence) Your higher self knows where you need to be.

TP: I keep getting the image of the same settlement burning down.

KL: It's burning down. So, what happened? Why is it burning down?

TP: I think an attack from another tribe or something.

KL: What's happening to the people in your community?

TP: They're either gone or about to leave. There are only one or two people left. They're trying to escape. I'm just there watching.

KL: Where is your family?

TP: They're not too far away from me.

KL: Is everybody ok?

TP: Yeah.

KL: Is there a name for your tribe?

TP: Akowa.

KL: Do you know which tribe attacked you? Are they still there, or are they gone?

TP: Some are there. I think they're looking around the place to see what they can take.

KL: Has this happened before?

TP: No.

KL: Do your tribe mix with other tribes?

TP: We've had some friendly encounters; so, to an extent, yes.

KL: So, what happens next? Where are your people, community, tribe going?

TP: I think they're going to go to another tribe that they've helped before so that they can have temporary help building up our own settlement again.

KL: Do you go with them? (Yeah) let's move forward; let's condense time and see what happens next.

TP: I see myself being forced into a ceremony; it's a traditional marriage ceremony.

KL: How old are you?

TP: I'm about 18; there's a guy from another tribe; it's not something I want to do.

KL: How are you feeling?

TP: I feel sad, trapped; it's not something I want to do. I just want to do my own thing and not have to follow the traditions.

KL: So, what stops you from doing your own thing?

TL: Fear that I'll be cast out and disappointing the family. It feels like there's an exchange, like a business deal, and if I don't do this, then the rest of the tribe and my family won't do as well as they could. So, I ended up going through with the arranged marriage. But I'm quite defiant. I still go off and do my own thing.

KL: What does your husband think of that?

TP: Annoyed, he doesn't like it. I think he wants me to be like the traditional quote-unquote wife, but I don't want to do that. I want to go out, travel, and explore.

KL: Does your husband not want to come with you?

TP: I don't want him to come. Not that I don't like him. It's just that I don't like that situation. If it were another guy, it would still be the same. It's not them specifically

KL: You like your independence. (Yeah.) Let's move forward and see what happens next.

TP: I feel like I'm doing something to do with fighting, or weapons training or something.

KL: What kind of weapons do you have?

TP: Bow and arrow; different kinds of swords.

KL: Are you good at fighting?

TP: Yes.

KL: How do you feel when you're fighting?

TP: A rush of adrenaline. It's powerful, agile. It's like I've got a purpose.

KL: Why are you learning to fight? Do women fight?

TP: It's not odd, but it's not the usual thing.

KL: Well, you're not the usual woman, are you. Let's move forward and see what happens next.

TP: I think we're going to war with another tribe? I'm not sure if it's the same one as before or a different one.

KL: How old are you now?

TP: Mid 20s. I want to go and join the fight, but my husband is opposed to it.

KL: What does he do?

TP: A carpenter possibly? I ended up going to fight, and he stayed. He's not happy, but he knows that I'm quite independent; if I'm going to do something, I'm going to do it.

KL: Yeah, he can't stop you. So, who do you fight with? Is there anything significant about their clothing that you notice?

TP: They've got fur.

KL: Do they have any markings on their face or their bodies? Do you have markings on your body? Things on your body?

TP: They have different hairstyles. Like something in the middle and then lines, I see three marks going down the cheek on either side

KL: What kind of marks? Is that their war paint?

TP: Yeah, I think it's more their tribal markings.

KL: Do you have any paint?

TP: On the arms, it's a thick band. Just the bands go around.

KL: What colour?

TP: Red, it's like a burgundy red.

KL: Do you have any marks on your face?

TP: Yes.

KL: And is this your tribal markings as well.

TP: Yes.

KL: What happens next?

TP: We are strategically laid out. I feel like I led this ambush and am given intel in terms of what way the other tribe is going to come and what strategies to take.

KL: How did you know?

TP: I tried to think like them, or if it were me and I was attacking this tribe, what would I do, what strategic offense I would take.

KL: So, the other people that are fighting with you, are they men or women?

TP: The majority are men. I don't think I can see any of the women at the moment.

KL: Do the men respect you?

TP: Yeah, I don't think there's any kind of animosity or anything.

KL: Is there any leader, or are you the leader?

TP: There is a leader, but he's very kind, understanding, and he listens; he's quite tall.

KL: Is he a good leader in this situation?

TP: Yes.

KL: What happens next? Let's move forward.

TP: I think we won that fight. There were a few casualties; it was a tough one.

KL: Do you go home?

TP: Yeah. We take all the casualties back to the settlement. I think I'm injured.

KL: Where are you injured?

TP: In the arm or shoulder? Yeah, like round here. (Pointing to the top of her arm/shoulder)

KL: Can you see what's happened?

TP: I think it's an internal injury.

KL: Okay. Let's move forward and see what happens.

TP: So, I'm in, like a witch doctor's hut, they're like the tribe's healer, and they've given me ointments, treatments for the neck and shoulder. I think it's a recurring thing, once every couple of days or once a week or something like that.

KL: What's happening now?

TP: I can't see anything at the moment, can't see anything past that.

KL: What can you feel? Is your shoulder better now?

TP: Yeah.

KL: Is there anybody else there with you? Where are you?

TP: Yeah, the living area.

KL: So, it's just you sat in the living room. How are you feeling?

TP: Content.

KL: Where's your husband?

TP: Making something.

KL: How do you feel about your husband now?

TP: He's there. He's just got on with it.

KL: Let's condense time and fast forward to the next significant time and see what's happening. Do you have children? What else happens in this lifetime?

TP: I think we've agreed to disagree and not have kids, and I think everyone else in the tribe is quite confused by that and disappointed. (laughing) That's something and one of the few things that we both agreed on. I see myself looking after other people's kids

KL: So, you like children then?

TP: Yeah.

KL: What made you decide not to have children of your own?

TP: I don't like the feeling of having to be constantly looking after someone else or something else and being trapped, and I like going off once in a while to explore.

KL: You like your freedom.

TP: Yeah. And if I were to go to war and I died, I don’t think it would be fair.

TP: I see myself in another war, and I think in this one I died.

KL: In the battle?

TP: In my 30s, mid-30s, and I think at this point I have become the leader.

KL: So, do you know who you were fighting?

TP: Just another tribe, we’ve been attacked. We don't go out and attack other tribes; it's always been that way. We haven't had many, but I think in this one, I died protecting someone else.

KL: Can you see who you’re trying to protect?

TP: Someone from my tribe who is fighting alongside me.

KL: And what happens in that fight? Who wins?

TP: We try to hold them up for as long as possible, but they win.

KL: So, what do your tribe do? Do they retreat?

TP: Yeah, they retreat.

KL: What's happened to your body?

TP: They've taken it.

KL: What's wrong with your body?

TP: A bow and arrow through the heart.

KL: So, what happens to you? You can see your body, but are you in your body?

TP: I'm looking down over my body.

KL: What do they do with the body?

TP: They take it back to the settlement and put me with the rest—with all the other people from the tribe who died in the battle.

KL: Were there many of you that died?

TP: There were a few of us. They bury our bodies, and they have a memorial.

KL: What happens next?

TP: There are people crying. Sad.

KL: How do you feel?

TP: Sad as well, but I've come to terms with it. Like I knew what I was getting into, I knew there was a chance of me dying, so I've already come to terms with death.

KL: So, what happens next?

TP: The rest of the people get on with their daily lives; they're upset, but you know.

KL: Is there anybody around you?

TP: My husband comes around and visits.

KL: Where are you?

TP: Somewhere on the astral plane.

KL: So, do you stay on the astral plane?

TP: Yeah, I just see myself watching over the tribe.

KL: Where did the other people go?

TP: They go to the next dimension when they're ready to go.

KL: Are you going to the next dimension?

TP: Eventually, yeah.

KL: Let's fast forward and see what happens. What's happening now?

TP: I can't see anything happening?

KL: So, do you go to the light?

TP: Yeah.

KL: Then what happens? Do you stay for a long time in the light?

TP: So, it's very warm. It feels easy and not filled with the stresses of life on earth.

KL: How long do you stay here in the light?

TP: I think for a while definitely. I think for a couple of years.

KL: It sounds like you deserve a little holiday. What happens next? Let's call your higher self in and ask why it's showing you that life and what the significance is with regard to this lifetime? Can I speak to your higher self?

TP: They showed me that because I am a fighter and a leader, and I'm not meant to go with the flow and do what's expected, or even if I do, I still can go against the grain, and it's okay to do that. I don't have to second guess myself.

KL: So, what does your higher self say about your purpose in this lifetime?

TP: I think it's to break barriers and boundaries. Not just for myself, but for other people.

KL: Yeah. And how will you do that?

TP: In my projects, by including people from under-represented backgrounds. The different areas of work that I'll go into or embark on for other people, I can do that, as well.

KL: Right? So, you're like breaking down stereotypes and inspiring other people to do what they choose to do.

TP: Yeah, yeah, exactly.

KL: So, not following the rules. So, what does your highest self say about your acting? Is there any guidance or advice that your higher self has for you in this lifetime now that you can create what you want to create?

TP: I think they're reassuring me that I'm on the right path and to just keep going and keep pushing. I'm not just going to do acting; there are other things that I will do as well that surround the creative industry.

KL: Great, and what other kinds of things will you do? Can you see?

TP: Filmmaking and directing.

KL: What does your higher self say regarding your concerns about not getting acting jobs?

TP: The jobs that I'm hoping for, they will come in. It's about divine timing. Just to be sure that I'm on the right path.

KL: Is there anything from the other life that needs to be resolved? Let's just ask your higher self to scan your body and see if there's anything from those lifetimes that needs resolving. How is your shoulder?

TP: I think it's not to be so complacent. There's nothing left they've got to say that I need to hear for the time being.

Reflections

My client found the session very interesting. She was amazed at the strength of the feelings and sensations in her body. She said that she could relate to and identify with a strong independent warrior spirit and fighting. She feels a strong sense of justice and a desire to fight for equality and the underdog in this life. She doesn't want children, though she enjoys looking after other people's children. 'It's like I won't be as free to do what I want to do, and plus, it's expensive. It's not cheap to raise kids, and it's quite a big responsibility.'

Her ambition as an actor is to give voice to marginalised people. She was grateful to connect with her higher self and reassured with the knowledge she was indeed on her soul path and to have faith in herself, her dreams, and her path. She will continue to develop her connection with her higher self.

Life Between Lives:

Soul Council Review

When a person dies, the soul leaves the physical body to return to source. Many clients in past life regression and in near-death experiences share similar experiences of going through the light, going through a tunnel, having a meeting with God or other light-beings or masters such as Jesus, Mother Mary, Buddha, Krishna, or a council of light. In the case of traumatic death, sometimes there is a healing and resting phase where the soul is healing and shedding any mental and/or emotional baggage before meeting with a 'Soul Council' for a life review. Before incarnating each Soul chooses themes for their life and what they want to experience and achieve, and soul contracts are put in place with others to allow for each person to experience and achieve what their soul desires. With the help of the soul council, they review their life. They get to see their lives and their interactions with others from a higher perspective and assess whether they achieved what they wanted to achieve and what they learned. Once you have completed the life review, you can then choose what to do and where to go next, depending on your life review. Some will stay and learn in the spirit realms and others may have a lifetime on other planets or reincarnate on the earth at some point. Many describe being given advice, guidance or options for life themes and also choosing the birth time, location, family, and physical body.

Pre-Conception Contracts

Pre-Conception Soul Contracts may be made with God, the Higher Self, or the Council or others before birth into the present life. Pre-Conception contracts can include;

a. Self-sacrifice or martyrdom for others

b. Teaching, leadership, or healing roles

c. Determining one's destiny

d. Learning particular lessons, or repaying karmic debts

e. Choices regarding family and parents

f. Patterns regarding health, illness, or death

These pre-conception contracts can often cause challenges and issues in life with relationships, health, work, business. What seemed like a good idea at the time of the life review and pre-conception contract may not be working so well for the personality on the Earth and it's possible to connect with the Higher Self and see if the soul contract can be changed or if there is another way to learn or resolve something. Many times, the soul is paying back a kindness from another lifetime or has made a vow in a past life to 'love someone forever' but the relationship isn't working out. If a soul wants to learn to have more compassion and be forgiving, they may create situations and experiences where they are betrayed or victimised to learn how to forgive others or they may need to learn how to forgive themselves. If the Higher Self agrees, the vow can be cleared and the pre-conception contracts can be changed or cancelled, or the Higher Self may have advice for the client with regard to their relationship or whatever areas of life where they are challenged. The higher self is a very loving and wonderful guide and resource to support us in creating a more conscious life and has a much fuller picture and higher perspective. As we mature and become more conscious, we embrace and embody more of our higher self.

Lord Asquith & The Americas:

Irina The Animal Healer & Celeste the Paramedic Angel

My client is an experienced healer and therapist and coach working in the field of mind, body, spirit. This was a 90-minute session, where my client went into a past life, life between life, another past life, and then into life between life, another past life and life in Spirit. Nearly all clients describe the death process and life between life in similar ways.

AR: I'm on a ship. It's like a big old-fashioned ship like The Onedin Line.

KL: Do you know where you're going?

AR: America or The Americas.

KL: Wow, the Americas, huh? Where are you coming from? Where were you travelling from before you got on the ship?

AR: Plymouth.

KL: Do you know the name of the ship?

AR: We call it the Mary Rose, but it's not really that; it's like a joke.

KL: Is there anything else about this ship that's significant or stands out for you?

AR: It's nearly all men, but there is a woman or some women.

KL: Are you male or female?

AR: I'm male.

KL: How old are you?

AR: Twenty-six?

KL: Can you look down at your feet and tell me what you're wearing?

AR: Black shoes, buckles on the shoes, stockings. Three-quarter length trousers. It's kind of like I'm meant to know what I'm doing, but I don't really. It's like I'm promoted above my level of ability.

KL: Okay, so are you working on the ship?

AR: Yeah, But I'll probably get off the other end and stay there. It's like I am, but I'm not.

KL: Ah, ok, what's your name?

AR: James.

KL: Well, hi, James. So, are you enjoying this trip?

AR: Not really, but kind of. The crew knows what they're doing, and I'm happy to tell them what to do, but they kind of know I don't really know what I'm doing. It's like because I'm from an aristocratic family, I get a higher rank, but I don't really know what I'm doing. So, I'm wary.

KL: I don't know too much about ranks, so are you Captain or what's your rank?

AR: No, like, First Officer. Okay.

KL: Yeah, so you're a little bit uncomfortable.

AR: A little bit, but I think I'm getting it. I know I'm getting off at the other end and staying there.

KL: Ok and what year is it?

AR: 1726.

KL: So, is there anything else significant about this moment, or shall we move forward?

AR: Yes, the sea's a little bit rough, not really rough, but there's water on my face.

KL: And how long does it take you to arrive in the Americas?

AR: We don't arrive.

KL: Ah. How long should it take?

AR: Six weeks, seven weeks.

KL: So, it's a long trip, but you don't arrive. Let's move forward to the next significant time and tell me what's happening now.

AR: We end up in the water.

KL: Do you know how you ended up in the water? What happened?

AR: I think, just a storm. I'm not sure. I'm not sure if everyone ended up in the water, but I did.

KL: Okay, so what happens next now that you're in the water?

AR: I'm just in the water holding onto a barrel. It's really cold, and there are other bits of wood and people. I think there are still people on the ship.

KL: How many people are there with you in the water?

AR: There are about twenty people in the water.

KL: Is there anybody there that you know?

AR: Not really. I don't really know anybody.

KL: Okay. So, you're holding onto the barrel, and it's really cold, what happens next? Is the ship coming back for you?

AR: No, it can't. There are no sails left now. I go under the water, but I end up in the sand. I lose the barrel, but when I wake up, I'm on the sand, it's warm. The sun is quite hot, not like boiling but warm.

KL: Do you know where you are?

AR: I want to say, Maine. New York. I don't know if it was Maine then or Maine now, but I want to say it's Maine now.

KL: What's it like there?

AR: There is like a kind of settlement, some people take me in, and they look after me. I'm not really ill; I'm tired, hungry, wet, and sunburnt and Mary is there.

KL: Who's Mary?

AR: A lady there in the settlement, and then she's, my wife.

KL: What's your life like with Mary? What do you do there in Maine?

AR: I feel bad because she's so good. She's so good. She doesn't complain. She doesn't want anything and never asks for anything, and it's kind of annoying. So, it's like, when I fell in love with her, it's because she was so pure, but it's kind of annoying because behind the purity, you can't reach her personality. She just is too good. There's no... I can't explain. It's like there's no personality. The fear of her thinking she's not good means she never expresses things. So, I get cross with her and hit her lots. And then I get cross with myself, and I really want to go to the city.

KL: What would the city give you?

AR: Money, women, alcohol, fighting, more gambling. More fun.

KL: So that's fun for you?

AR: Yeah.

KL: What about Mary?

AR: Yeah, I feel bad. It's like I thought she was my salvation, and she just makes me annoyed because it's not me. You can't teach someone to be good. They just are or they aren't.

KL: Do you have any children?

AR: Yes, she's got one in her belly now, but I want to go. I think I'll go.

KL: Okay, so where do you go? What happens next?

AR: New York. She won't find me. People will look after her. It's okay.

KL: Did you tell her you were going?

AR: No. I am selfish and spoiled and arrogant, and I don't care.

KL: So now you're in New York, are there lots of women?

AR: There are, but they're dirty, though.

KL: In what way?

AR: No washing. Disease. But I'll get a rich wife here. They like my voice, and they like my title.

KL: What's your title?

AR: Lord.

KL: What's your surname James?

AR: Asquith.

KL: And where did you live? I'm curious. Where did you live before you set sail from Plymouth?

AR: Yorkshire. My father told me to go because I'm in trouble.

KL: What happened that got you into trouble?

AR: Gambling. He told me to go and make a new life. So, I have the same life in a new place.

KL: So, are you gambling in New York?

AR: Yes, they like me here.

KL: Where do you get the money to gamble?

AR: It's fine; it's my inheritance, my trust fund.

KL: So, you're in contact with your mum and dad?

AR: Yes. But it's my bank. Name and reputation go a long way.

KL: So, what do you do in New York?

AR: Parties, dancing, feud, and the odd duel, but it's more for fun. But I did shoot him in the knee.

KL: Who did you shoot?

AR: Another man, I thought if he shoots first, I'll see what happens, but I shot first. I didn't want to kill him. I shot him.

KL: Then what happens?

AR: (Laughing) Hurt him. He's okay; he's got a stick now.

KL: You must be very good friends!

AR: I was drunk. It was a joke. We were drunk. It was a duel. It's all gentlemanly.

KL: So, let's move forward to the next significant time in your life.

AR: I have the pox now. I'm dying of Syphilis.

KL: How old are you now?

AR: I'm 43.

KL: You're quite young.

AR: I've had a good life, lots of fun. I'm not so young.

KL: So, how do you die? What happens?

AR: I'm just in bed; there are people there. A nurse and a woman fussing. It's okay. I'm ready to die. Damn pain in my head, though. Like a worm.

KL: So, let's move forward to when you die and leave your body; what happens next? AR: I seem to be floating about. I know I'm meant to go up, but I don't. I quite like flying about like someone in a long nightdress; it's fun. I know I'm meant to go up, but I really want to see what it's like to fly about.

KL: Why is it such fun flying about?

AR: It's really free. It's like, yeah,

KL: Yes, free, free as a bird. So, where do you go when you're flying about?

AR: Yeah. It's just like a night sky. And it's like, you know when you go up, there's kind of roles and responsibilities. And when you're down there, there are roles and responsibilities. And this is like the only place when you're totally free, but it gets boring. So, then you go up eventually. I'm gonna go up now. As you go up, you start being bathed in light, and it feels like being frozen in light. I guess like a statue. It's like it re-programs you, like washing or something, and I have the sensation of 'here we go again.' I have this sort of sensation of I know I'm meant to learn virtues, learn how to be good, and I kind of know how to do that, so I'm kind of more interested in seeing how bad you can be.

KL: So, what did you learn from that lifetime?

AR: More finding about that human concept of bad but not really bad. Not like hurting people; just like not following the conventional rules.

KL: You don't like the rules?

AR: The rules were boring, and then, like then, they were stupid. If you want to eat, if you want to drink, great! It's your money; if you want to gamble, gamble. Who cares? It's not like you're hurting anybody.

KL: How did your parents feel when you had to leave to start a new life?

AR: Mother never says anything anyway. My father is all about reputation. And that's stupid. It's hypocrisy. I'd rather be real to me than be a hypocrite like him.

KL: So, when you left, did you have gambling debts?

AR: Yeah, but I had the money to pay them. Mm-hmm. So, they were paid. It's more the scandal. He doesn't like the scandal. If I didn't have any money, I wouldn't do it. It's my money. I can do what I want.

KL: So, what are you going to do now?

AR: I'm waiting. I'm having a think. My Soul is re-creating. My memories going. Happy, joyful soul. All pretty and ready to go.

KL: Ready to go where?

AR: I can go anywhere I want. I can choose.

KL: Is there anyone else with you?

AR: Yeah. All in their own spaces, ready to choose.

KL: So how do you choose when you can go anywhere?

AR: I wait for inspiration; sometimes, we talk about it - get ideas off each other. Sometimes, some of the souls just disappear, like they chose and went, or they got taken to go. We pretend we're frightened that they got taken to go, but we know we choose ourselves. It's like a kind of mock horror, like, 'Oh no, we've been taken!' We know they chose, and I feel like I'm digging my heels in a bit and don't want to choose yet. I feel like I'm fighting with myself. I feel like I should learn some virtues in a struggling way. I don't know why I think I should. But I kind of want to have a fun, joyful, easy life. Well, then I'm torn because I get bored if it's too easy. I don't want pain, hardship, or poverty. I want ease. I'm struggling to work out how to make it interesting. I think I need to learn, and this is weird because this is what I talk to my clients about all the time. I think I need to learn that it can be easy, it can be fun. And you can learn and be challenged through creating more rather than battling through a struggle. So maybe I need to do that. But I'm kind of considering that now and thinking yeah, but if I do that, I might create mischief.

KL: You have a naughty side, huh?

AR: So, I stay until I decide what to do.

KL: So, let's move forward to the time that you choose.

AR: So, it kind of worked out then through positive creation... struggle... and so I heal animals. I'm very good. And it's so weird because I'm really good, but she was beautiful and kind. But she was really good. Part of me is sneering at that choice. It's so weird. But the positive learning – that's fun. But also creating rather than struggling. Healing animals with touch, and having really good, telepathic communication with the light. They just come to me, and I can heal their wounds. I'm touching them or putting my hand over them, and I can heal their minds by looking into their eyes. And it's really nice to be able to do that.

KL: So, does it make you happy doing that?

AR: Yeah. And it brings me a lot of peace, and I guess satisfaction.

KL: You don't get bored?

AR: No, I feel very content. It was a good choice that night.

KL: So, how old are you now in this life?

AR: I'm about seventeen.

KL: Excellent. So, are you living with your family?

AR: Yes and no, I don't know what that means.

KL: Okay, what's your name?

AR: Irina.

KL: Irina, do you have any siblings?

AR: Yes, there are 12 of us.

KL: 12 of you, gosh.

AR: Yeah, some are not complete brothers and sisters, but we are brothers and sisters. The little one is the son of the big brother, but he's like a little brother because his wife died. Okay, so we're not real brothers and sisters, but we like to be part of such a big family. Sometimes It's hard because my big brother acts like my dad. My dad's very gentle. My big brothers are very protective, and I'm not sure how this protective behaviour helps me; you know, he doesn't like me. He likes to know where I am, and he doesn't want me to have a suitor. He'd like me to take money for healing the animals, but I don't.

KL: So where are you living right now?

AR: In a wooden house, like a little chalet. My dad is here, but he's sick, he's quite old. My mom lives in the house here.

KL: Let's move forward to the next significant time. How old are you now?

AR: 24. I'm about to get married to Hans. I did want to marry him to be happy.

KL: What does Hans do?

AR: He's a woodcutter; he cuts trees that give people firewood which keeps the forest thinned. He brings me animals sometimes when they get hurt. When we were children, he used to throw things at me to get my attention.

KL: So, you've known him a long time.

AR: Since we were five. Now he's big and handsome. He was my boyfriend in this lifetime.

KL: Ah! Let's move forward and see what happens next.

AR: We have a baby. She died, she was too sick, and I couldn't make her better.

KL: How old was your baby?

AR: Just five or eight months old.

KL: What was her name?

AR: Hannah. I should have been able to make her better because I could make animals better, but I couldn't because she was just sick all the time. I'm not a good healer.

KL: That's what you decided?

AR: That's what Hans told me because I can make animal wounds disappear with my hands. I should be able to make a baby stop being sick. I couldn't. It was like she wanted to go because we tried everything. She was teaching me about free will, okay. That's a hard pill to swallow. Hans and I were learning about love, but we didn't learn it because we were never happy after that.

KL: What happens next?

AR: I don't know if I thought he blamed me or he really did blame me. It was like living in a house with someone, but it's not a marriage. It's like living, just being polite in a curt way, and everybody thinks everything's okay. Because if it is in public, you're polite, but in the house, it's like two strangers living together. And I can't heal animals very well now. It's not the same. It's like I've lost my touch.

KL: So, let's move forward to the next significant time.

AR: I have a son now; he's eight.

KL: Is this Hans' son?

AR: Yes.

KL: What do you call your son?

AR: Pete. He likes to go out with his father. There is no relationship really between my husband and me now. He's just my husband. We didn't learn about that.

KL: How do you feel?

AR: I feel sad. I really want to know how to get my healing abilities back. But I think it's something to do with learning about love. But I don't know how to do that with him anymore. I don't feel connected, but I don't know what to do. And I'm hardly healing the wounded animals now, with my hands. Sometimes they get better eventually, but I used to be able to do it instantly. And other times they get better when we use poultices. And sometimes like I know it's connected to the relationship or not learning, but I don't know. I can't learn about it with Hans because he doesn't want to. It has to be together like an agreement, and he's not trying.

KL: So, let's move forward again. Let's fast forward to the next significant time.

AR: And I live on my own now. Hans has married a woman in another village now. But I look quite young still, so people say I'm a witch because I look younger than I am.

KL: So, where are you living now?

AR: In a small house cottage. I'm older now. I'm 71 now, but I look 60. Yeah, my hair is too yellow. My skin has not really aged much.

KL: Really! Can you tell us your secret?

AR: I feel it's a blessing. I'm blessed with youth and beauty, I guess.

KL: what happens next?

AR: Oh, I made lots of poultices and things like mashing up things to put on wounds for animals and liquid remedies for people. They're not instant anymore, but they do help. And then I taught myself all about plants from just trial and error. It's like healing with my hands is almost like a dream, like, 'Was that real?' but I know it was.

KL: Now you work with the herbs and the plants?

AR: Yeah, I put my hands on sometimes, I have, like an instinct, but it's almost like I know it's not going to heal instantly as it did before, and of course, it doesn't. But animals still like me; they come right up to the door like in a fairy tale—you know, rabbits, birds, deer, foxes, and that sort of thing. Like a badger and there are fairies too. Don't tell anyone. There are fairies on the windowsill.

KL: I won't tell. Sounds like a nice little family.

AR: Yeah.

KL: Like a little fairy tale family. What's happening now?

AR: I think I'm dead. I just fall asleep before another life, and I know when I'm lying in my bed. I know I'm not going to wake up, and that's fine, and the animals are coming in. It's like they're watching after me so that I don't feel alone, which is returning a kindness. I guess we know we 'get' each other.

KL: Let's move forward to when you leave your body.

AR: Just leaving, you tumble about a bit which makes you feel a bit sick, and then you just go straight up. Ready to go. It looks like a separate place. I'm floating and getting washed, but this time it feels more like rinsing off in a separate place. So, the lights just coming through me and it's part of me, and I'm feeling just like a little speck of glitter. I'm not the whole ocean of creator, so I can see myself as a separate glitter, but the whole creation is glitter.

KL: So, what do you do?

AR: Well, you're just completely restful and wonderful, and you can stay here as long as you like. It's like a massive recharge. Then when I come back, I'm going to be, not told, but suggested or asked, if this would be a good path for me. I can be an angel, but this type is more like a paramedic angel. So, it's kind of like you're hanging out with the emergency first aid kit. And then, if someone needs you, you attend to them.

KL: Oh, that sounds interesting. How does that work?

AR: Oh, I don't know. Say they're in a car crash or something, and you attend to them; if they call you or someone calls you. Then you get back up to the staff room and wait to be called again. It's like a paramedic. It's cool. It's kind of fun in the staff room. Sometimes it can be tiring because you could be on a long shift. But it's always so amazing to be able to help someone.

KL: Do you ever feel sad?

AR: No, because I know what I'm doing, and it's like a request. Somebody prays for you or asks for you, or somebody else asks for you, and then the light goes on. Or, and then one of you goes, unless it's sometimes, you know, it's, you're the best one for the job or, sometimes you know, someone else is the best one for the job. Oftentimes, you're the only one there, so you have to; it's kind of like that, but not sad. I mean, everybody is choosing right.

KL: And so, do you have a name? What do people call you?

AR: Celeste.

KL: So, do you have friends in the staff room?

AR: We're all friends. It's not like a human relationship. But we're all friends.

KL: Okay, sometimes you work on your own. Do you ever work together on things?

AR: Sometimes, we work together. I think if it's like an earthquake or something or a famine.

KL: So, what do you do if there's an earthquake?

AR: Sometimes people think they came out of holes on their own, but they really don't. You kind of push them up or make a bridge or make yourself look like a ledge or a foot hole. So, they'll say, I don't know how I did it, but I climbed 'out' and yet they can... And then yeah, and sometimes humans are like ants. They work so hard to like, move a few stones to get people out, but they're really not strong enough. So sometimes, we work alongside them, and they don't know. Sometimes they can see us. Yeah, sometimes they can see us, and they'll say to others, and some believe them and sometimes that's okay. Sometimes you're just staying in the dark, endless space with a person who's trapped, so they don't feel alone.

KL: That's kind.

AR: It doesn't feel like I'm being kind. It's just they pray for you, and you go; that's a job. We don't try to be kind. That's just the way we are. It's a job. All of you can't do this job. If you don't know, those virtues. If you haven't mastered them, you can't do that job. This is not a job to learn stuff. This is a job to not even practice. It's just a job that has to be done by some of us, and you have to have the right qualification. So, does that make sense? It's a life of service. Yes, yeah. You enjoy it. Yeah. You have fun.

KL: So, let's move forward to the next significant time.

AR: I'm gonna be swapped out. It's like I've done enough. I feel a little, little sad because I felt like I could have gone on longer. I've had fun, and I'm happy. I kind of would like to have stayed longer, but I'm not sure why I have to be swapped out. I think it's just, it's time for someone else to have that experience, and you only need so many. I asked him. I said, 'Do I have to leave?' And that's what they said. Someone else needs the experience, and you've got lots of experience now as you've been here the longest. So, you're gonna stop doing it now.

KL: Do you know where you'll go next?

AR: I get to have a chat with someone and swept aside with someone who's maybe a bit like be a counsellor. So, I can think about what I want. But I think I feel it's probably a good idea to do another human one now.

KL: Do you want to do that? Do you want to continue and see what's next? Or do you feel like you've done enough today? What would you like to do?

AR: I can just tell you what I'm gonna do. And so, I think in this kind of chat with this 'counsellor' about... Okay, what's next? I'll do a human one. And then as soon as we talked about... Yeah, I should probably do a human one. Straightaway. I'm like, okay, I'm gonna have loads of money this time cos I know money is like a key. And it's pretty crap not having money, so I'm gonna make sure I have loads. I think I want to practice playing with money. Hmm. You know, like having loads to start with, creating more, learning about alchemy. That's what I'm gonna do.

KL: That sounds fun. Yeah. So maybe we can look at that another time. So, let's ask your higher self to tell us why you've been given these lifetimes what the relevance is to your current life.

AR: I know I don't think the first one. I don't know; maybe I always know that I've had lifetimes because I know I can read the stars. So maybe it was just to show me another one.

KL: Let's call in your higher self and ask your higher self. So just relax, and let's invite your higher self to come forward. Let's speak to your higher self and get some clarification to see why they have shown you these lifetimes.

AR: It was something to do with the balance and understanding the difference between being yourself and being what other people expect you to be. M-hmm and understanding that on a human level, there are conventions and rules depending on cultures. And you can choose to abide by them or if they don't seem right for you, you can choose to look somewhere else where the conventions and rules are different, or go somewhere where there is nobody, and make your own. But you do have to recognise that man creates these conventions, and you can choose to fit in, move on or break them. There would be consequences not from the creator but by man. Yeah.

KL: And so why do you think it is important for Annie to see that?

AR: I have no idea.

KL: Is there someone there that knows?

AR: I don't have... I genuinely don't.

KL: So, is that of significance to Annie's current life?

AR: The only thing is with clients. I mean, like you, I have clients all over the world, and you know, you have to get in and you can't go straight into it. Well, this is your free will;

you're choosing to create something different because they are so bound by their cultural conventions or traditions. Maybe it's just a reminder to not go in too deep too soon when they cannot comprehend the soul concepts. That's the only thing I can think of.

KL: Is there anybody in those lifetimes that you recognise as being with you in this lifetime?

AR: So, Hans was one last boyfriend. The baby was my daughter; the lesson was about free will, to teach me that if somebody dies, it's that they choose their death. The soul is free. It doesn't mean that you're not good at healing or you're not good enough. The lesson was that we all have free will.

KL: Yeah. So, do you have that lesson in this lifetime?

AR: Yeah, I thought so, but obviously, I needed reminding. If I think of other people who I'm close to in my life, I get it. But if I think of Sammy, I don't get it. It's like I always feel she's doing it for the greater good. She's not totally choosing free will. She's doing it because she thinks it would be best for someone else or it's for the best. Yeah, I kind of feel she doesn't have complete free will; she always tries to think about what is best for someone would be. Maybe I need to learn that even if it is best for someone else that she's still got free will, and that's something she's got to learn.

KL: Yeah. Well, maybe if you learn it, she'll get it too. We know how things pass down through the ancestral line. So, would you like to bring forward all the virtues and all the lessons or blessings again, from each of these lifetimes, everything that you've learned and that serves you? Maybe bringing forward those gifts and abilities of the animals and the instant healing and remembering that everybody has free will, including the animals, and everybody can choose. That you can heal instantly if the people are ready to be healed instantly that sometimes they might be choosing to move on and that's ok.

AR: Yeah.

KL: Is there anything else that you want to bring forward?

AR: Yeah, I think it's about releasing that doubt because when I couldn't heal a baby, then I lost faith in myself and in the possibilities, and the miracles, and my own abilities.

KL: So, let's release any fear, any doubt, any kind of feeling like you're not good enough or you can't heal anymore. And let's teach you on all levels that you know how to be able to heal instantly if people are ready to be healed instantly. And that sometimes that healing is actually assisting them in their transition. And that you don't need to doubt yourself or feel bad about your abilities because it's up to them and the creator. Can we remove any fear that you have around Sammy or any of your children so that you can be relaxed and know that you're always aware if you're required to assist them at any point without needing to be worried or concerned or frightened for them?

AR: Yes, all of that.

KL: So, anything else that you want to bring forward?

AR: The Alchemy.

KL: From the next lifetime, you mean? (Yeah.) Okay. Let's ask that you can have that now, and I wonder if you might want to bring forward that blessing of youth and beauty.

AR: Yes, that would be great.

KL: Yeah, that's pretty amazing. Let's bring that forward. So, you know what it feels like to be blessed with youth and beauty and that you have this in this life now. And I wonder what you're learning in this lifetime that's connected with these two lifetimes. There seems to be a kind of a theme around love.

AR: I think the first one was learning to choose someone who's not someone who can teach you stuff or because you think they have certain qualities and they'll kind of rub off on you, or to be infatuated because they have certain qualities, but rather to choose someone who's got the same values as you. And then the second one must have been about communication because it surely could have been repaired through honest communication. I also think on the second one, it was like, I think I did try to communicate but he couldn't or wouldn't, and I should have realized, rather than be lonely, to have loved myself enough to ...okay I don't think you could be separated then but to completely live my own life, and not feel that because he wasn't able to communicate and shut himself off, that therefore I had to be diminished.

This session was integrated using direct suggestion and Theta Healing energy healing with the positive beliefs and feelings downloaded into the client's unconscious mind and cellular memory and through all time, space, dimension, and reality.

KL: So, let's teach you, and remind you of that, you know how and what it feels like that you're always able to be all of who you are, no matter who or what anybody else is choosing, that it's easy for you to be yourself and to be all of who you are. You know how to communicate and to be without diminishing yourself no matter what anyone else is choosing. So, would you like to know that those lessons are completed, so that you can be free to choose somebody you can share the love with, in the way that you choose? That you can be happy and content yourself and that you can be happy and content with somebody else and share your life with someone else? It's possible.

AR: Yes.

KL: So, is there anything else that needs to be integrated?

AR: No.

KL: Is there anybody else in those lifetimes that you're connected with now in this lifetime?

AR: I think my father in the first one was my father in this one. I think maybe my son was in the second life, and some of us were angels at the same time. Maybe that's how we do it in soul families.

Reflections

The client was amazed at the amount of detail they experienced and how the session went from the past life to a life between life and then into another past life etc. The client has recently started dating, so perhaps this is why the higher self chose to focus on the theme of love and relationships.

A week or so after this session I was amazed to see a BBC new story of an emergency paramedic angel flying through the air with a jetpack to a remote mountain location to rescue someone. I'm sure flying with our angelic wings is a much easier way to travel, but it was wonderful to once again see the synchronicities that show up on this path.

Great American Depression & World War 2:

Life Between Lives – Soul Contracts – Choices – Timelines

This client has only ever done one past life regression with another hypnotherapist, where she only got vague information and so was interested to take part in this project. In this session we go into two past lives and a life between lives, exploring the life review process, soul contracts and the choices and possibilities available to choose from before incarnating.

LJ: I see children, there are a few, but one little girl stands out more than the other. She's wearing a red dress and pigtails too, and she's got a round, happy face.

KL: Does she look familiar?

LJ: She feels familiar.

KL: How do you think this little girl is connected to you?

LJ: She's maybe eight or nine. There are lots of other children, but she's in front of everybody else. She's jumping up and down as though to try to get my attention. She's really pleased to see me; she hasn't seen me for a long time, and she's so excited and happy.

KL: So, where are you? Take a moment to look around and see what's around you.

LJ: It's a wide-open space, quite flat. Initially, it's quite flat, but further into the distance, there are mountains in the background, but they seem a long way away. There's no snow on them. So, it feels very warm. I feel I'm somewhere warm. There are massive fields of golden wheat or corn or maize or some crop. There are swathes of it all around and there doesn't seem to be any end to it.

KL: Wonderful. And does this little girl have a name?

LJ: Eloise. She wants to take me by the hand. She wants to take me inside this house. It's a very lovely house; it's a simple house, just one storey. She's very keen to have me go inside and look around. It's very plain, not painted or anything. Everything is made of wood. Everything's clean; it's all very plain. There's nothing fancy about it. There's a lovely feeling in this house—friendly, very friendly. I have this wonderful sense of being home and belonging, surrounded by family. The feeling is coming up through my body. There's lots of love, and there's space and time for everybody. Yeah, even though there are a lot of people associated with the house, there has always been enough for everybody. There's not a lack of anything. Not masses, but just plentiful—plentiful love, plentiful time. There's a lovely feeling of quality about everything but not lavish or luxurious. It's quite simple.

KL: So, just taking a moment to look down at your feet. Can you see your feet?

LJ: I've got some leather sandals on. I'm male.

KL: And how old are you?

LJ: 40.

KL: What are you wearing?

LJ: Long, long waistcoat and short trousers that go to my ankles.

KL: I should have asked your name before I asked what you're wearing.

LJ: My name is John, but I'm called Jack.

KL: And so, Jack, who is Eloise?

LJ: She's my first little girl.

KL: And is this your house?

LJ: Yes, this is my home. Mm-hmm. I built it.

KL: You built it. Wow! Sounds amazing. I love wood. So, tell me, Jack, is your wife there?

LJ: Not anymore; there's a presence of her, but I can't find her here.

KL: So, is there anybody else that lives there with you?

LJ: I have some sons here, but they're much older.

KL: How many sons do you have?

LJ: I have two, but I had three. I had three sons, but now I have two.

KL: Oh, what happened to your other son?

LJ: He got sick, and we're a long way from getting any help, so we just do what we can.

KL: I'm sorry. Where are you living? What country is this?

LJ: It's America.

KL: Is it a particular part of America?

LJ: Montana. We live at the bottom; we don't live up in the hills. We can see the hills from where we are.

KL: And what year is it?

LJ: 1906.

KL: So, what's happening now? It's you and Eloise, and you said you've got two other sons. Do these other sons live with you in the house?

LJ: Yes, they live here. It's a big house; there's room for everybody in the house.

KL: And what do you do?

LJ: I farm. This is my crop.

KL: What do you grow?

LJ: I grow wheat.

KL: Wheat. Mm-hmm. That's a beautiful crop, the golden crop. Do you have animals? Cattle?

LJ: No cattle, just crop.

KL: What do your sons do? Do they work with you?

LJ: We work together. They work on the farm with me. One day it will be their farm.

KL: Not for a while.

LJ: No, not for a while (laughs).

KL: So, let's condense time and let's move forward to the next significant time and see what happens.

LJ: I have a great weight on my chest. It feels like I'm having difficulty breathing.

KL: Do you know what's wrong with your body?

LJ: No. There's something in my lungs. It's okay. I'm not afraid.

KL: You're not afraid of what?

LJ: It's my time to leave this world. That's what's going to happen. My sons will have the farm, and they will bring their families. It will all be theirs, and life will go on and my life will go on through them.

KL: And how old are you now, Jack?

LJ: I'm 65.

KL: So, Eloise is grown up now?

LJ: Yes.

KL: Do you have grandchildren?

LJ: Yes, but they're very tiny.

KL: How old are your sons?

LJ: They're older; my sons are in their 40s now. I have only one of them here, he has a beautiful wife, and she lives with us, and she helps. They look after me.

KL: That's wonderful. What are your sons called?

LJ: One's called John after me, and the other is called Joshua. Now we couldn't call him Jack because they call me Jack.

KL: So, Joshua and John. Beautiful. So, what happens next?

Client now moves into a life between lives experience.

LJ: I'm going to join my wife.

KL: Wonderful.

LJ: It's a good day. She's waiting for me.

KL: How does she look?

LJ: Very beautiful, long, golden hair.

KL: Just as you remember her?

LJ: Yes, when I first met her.

KL: What's your wife's name?

LJ: Ruth.

KL: So, you meet Ruth and then what happens?

LJ: I'm in a white space. It's hard to see, though it seems very misty now like there's a cloud almost.

KL: Just take a breath and allow the space to clear so that you can see clearly.

LJ: I must go through this tunnel faster. There are lots of people wanting to come as well, but they can't come.

KL: Do you know any of those people in the tunnel?

LJ: No, but they want my help, they're asking to come with me, but it's not their time yet. They must wait.

KL: Do those people have bodies?

LJ: Sort of, but not like real bodies.

KL: Do you have a body?

LJ: Not anymore. I don't need a body anymore.

KL: They need to shift their bodies first, right? Okay, so what happens next?

LJ: I can see what looks like a lecture theatre. Mm-hmm. It's the same people, but they're not people. They're like energies, and they have a form, but they don't have clear faces. They are translucent. They're asking me to tell them everything I've done, and they want to see if I've fulfilled my contract to see whether I can go through the next door.

KL: So, what do they say about your contract? Are they talking about your soul contract?

LJ: It's my sole purpose on earth.

KL: What was your purpose in that lifetime?

LJ: They have a list, and they're going through this list. They want to know if I tithed some of my earnings to help other people, and I did that. Was I a good man? I think I was a good man. I brought my sons up after my wife passed away. I didn't think there was a contract. I had a good life. There was lots of love in the home, and the doors were always open to other people.

KL: So, what do these beings decide about your contract?

LJ: They're happy. So, there are two doors. I can choose if I want to have another contract, and they'll lay out the terms of that contract. But I won't know all the terms of the contract when I make a choice, or I can choose to move on. They're asking me if I feel I have unfinished and unresolved things that I would like to explore in another lifetime. They said this is an opportunity if I want to grow more, because on the other side of the other door, there are other levels, and if I go through that, then I could be on one level. If I come back and have another contract, then I could come in at a higher level. It's not easy to make a choice because you don't know the answers. I had a good life. Maybe I could have another good life. Then again, I'm curious to know what's on the other side.

KL: Can you get a sense of what's on the other side of each of those doors?

LJ: Both doors are slightly open.

KL: Can you feel which one is pulling you more?

LJ: I just think if I go back at this point, it may not be a good idea because that's looking quite dark. You must go back through the tunnel. It could be quite exciting to go back again this time. I can't decide. How can I decide? Okay, some other people are coming forward, and they're saying to me if you take that contract, we will come with you. They say they'll come with me, that they'll meet up with me, and they will help me fulfil that contract.

KL: Do you know these people?

LJ: Yes, I feel I know them. But I don't know. I don't know.

KL: Is Ruth there?

LJ: Yes, but she's not going to come back this time. She says that's fine, but it wouldn't be her contract.

KL: So, what do you choose?

LJ: I'm going back for another lifetime. I must go back through the tunnel. You forget what will come. It's like, wait, that's not how that works! How are you ever going to work it out? It's so frustrating to remember what was on the contract. But I know I have these people who are going to be with me, and I just must find them. I must find them, and they will help me fulfil that contract.

The client now moves forward into another life.

KL: So, let's move forward in time and take a nice deep breath. Let's condense time. Let's see what happens next.

LJ: I'm in a very noisy city.

KL: Can you describe the city?

LJ: Lots of tall buildings. Lots of noise.

KL: Just take a moment to look down at your feet. What are you wearing on your feet?

LJ: I've got very smart shoes on.

KL: What's the shape?

LJ: They're brown leather lace-up shoes with pointy toes.

KL: What else are you wearing?

LJ: I'm wearing a smart suit with a very sharp crease down the front of my trousers.

KL: Wonderful. What's your name? What do people call you?

LJ: Alan.

KL: Hi, Alan. So, you've got a smart suit, wonderful pointy shoes, that sounds very cool. Where do you work?

LJ: I work in the city bank.

KL: Which bank do you work for?

LJ: The National Bank of America.

KL: The National Bank of America, that's fantastic, and have you always wanted to work in a bank?

LJ: No, but it was a good job. You must take a job somehow.

KL: How old are you now, Alan?

LJ: Mm-hmm, I'm 30.

KL: Do you have a family?

LJ: I have a mother, but she's very frail. Hmm. And I must support her.

KL: Do you live with your mother?

LJ: She lives with me. Mm-hmm. We have a cat.

KL: What's your cat called?

LJ: Toby. It's my mother's cat, really.

KL: Do you like cats? Was it your cat or your mother's cat?

LJ: My cat, but now he's my mother's cat. She makes a fuss about him.

KL: You mentioned that your mother was frail. What's wrong with your mother?

LJ: She's just very elderly.

KL: How old is your mother?

LJ: She must be in her 60s, but her hips aren't good.

KL: It's nice that you look after her.

LJ: It's ok, we bob along. I help her. My father left us a long time ago.

KL: Oh, what happened?

LJ: It was a long time ago. Mm-hmm. I don't remember much about it.

KL: Do you have any other brothers or sisters?

LJ: No.

KL: So, it's just you and your mom. So, let's condense time and let's move forward to a significant time and tell me what's happening.

LJ: It's in the paper.

KL: What's in the paper?

LJ: There's been a crash on Wall Street. Everybody's going to lose their money. I'm not going to have a job. This is going to be tough. What am I going to do?

KL: Is your mum still living with you?

LJ: Okay, we'll manage or can't see how we're going to manage. She says it's more important to help other people than to help ourselves. I say, how are you going to do that when you haven't got any money? She says that's not important. It's what's in your heart that's important.

KL: Is your mom religious?

LJ: Yes, she is.

KL: What's your mother's religion?

LJ: She's Jewish, but she's not been able to go to the synagogue for a long time because she's not well enough.

KL: Do you go to the synagogue?

LJ: No.

KL: What do you think about religion?

LJ: It's a waste of time.

KL: What makes you think that?

LJ: Well, if there were a God, there wouldn't be so much bad stuff going on.

KL: What kind of stuff?

LJ: People fighting, poverty, sadness, my dad leaving, all that crap. If there was a God, he'd be looking out for us. Mm-hmm.

KL: You have to look out for yourself.

LJ: Yeah. I have to look out for myself, and I have to look out for my mom.

KL: So, what happens next?

LJ: So, I'm in a hall, it's like a place at the town hall where you go, and people can get fed, and I go there and help them. I volunteer. But also, I go and see if I can get other food, get people to contribute food so that people who really have nothing can get fed.

KL: Do you enjoy that?

LJ: Well, it's a good thing to do, and I don't have a job right now, so I'm contributing in that way. That's okay. It means I get fed too at some point. My mom's not here anymore.

KL: Oh, what happened to your mum?

LJ: She just took up and died.

KL: I'm sorry to hear that.

LJ: She had her religion; she was fine. I have this family here now, with all these people. Everybody is helping each other.

KL: It sounds like a nice little community there.

LJ: Yes, they're sharing, and they don't have much, but they're happy to share what they have.

KL: How old are you now, Alan?

LJ: I think 47.

KL: So, what's happening in the economy?

LJ: It's still tough. It's still tough for people.

KL: You never went back to banking?

LJ: No. I didn't want to do what I was doing anyway.

KL: If you could do anything, what would you like to do?

LJ: Do you know what would be nice? It would be to get a house and to take in all the children who don't have families, give them a better life, educate them, and feed them and clothe them. That would be a good thing. That's what I really would like to do. So maybe just being able to help with this food and ensure people are fed, maybe something will come about. Maybe there'll be an opportunity. Hmm.

KL: Does that make you happy?

LJ: Yeah, that would make me very happy. I don't have a wife or a girl. Just think that children need somebody. Oh, I could be a dad without being a father. Mm-hmm.

KL: How do you feel about women?

LJ: I'm not so bothered. They're pretty, but I'm not bothered.

KL: So, let's move forward and see what happens.

LJ: I see a church.

KL: What type of church?

LJ: Big church, very imposing. There are these guys wearing long black coats, with something white around them and they're connected to this church. I'm with them, but I'm not wearing those clothes.

KL: So, you said it was long black cloaks with something white around them?

LJ: Long black cloaks, like dresses, with a white cord around the middle.

KL: What are you doing at the church?

LJ: They said they would house the children, and it's nice they want to house the children, but I want to make sure it's going to be good for the children. I don't know because I'm not a religious person, but these guys are religious. I don't know if that's a good thing or a bad thing. But if it's a way to house the children, maybe we just need to go along with that. There are lots of orphans of all ages. They need a good meal, some of them you see them on the street, and they beg, and I just want to gather them all up and bring them in and keep them safe.

KL: Let's move forward and see what happens.

LJ: I am in a school. I teach the children in this place.

KL: Uh-huh. What do you teach them?

LJ: Just basic stuff. I'm not really a teacher. How to read and do maths.

KL: How old are the children?

LJ: Some are quite small, maybe eight or nine. Some are in their teens. They're not so keen on learning, but they do; they're good kids, really.

KL: So where do these children live?

LJ: There's a place next to the church where they live. They must share rooms, and they must bunk up together, but it's ok, it's clean, and it's warm.

KL: So, who looks after the children? Do you live with them?

LJ: Well, no, I don't live there. I just go, and I keep an eye on everything. And the people who help are those I met before, and they come, and they help. They make sure that the children are fed, and I just go, and I teach school.

KL: So, are these people who look after the children the people in the long black cloaks? The religious people?

LJ: No, they're all ladies who come to help. And there's one lady she lives there, and she's good. She's a good one. Annie. The children love her. We have about 15 children. We could take more if we had space. One day, maybe.

KL: And how do you find the money to look after these children?

LJ: People bring us donations, or they bring us clothes or books. We don't always necessarily have physical money, though. We have people who give us things. They donate to the church, and then the church brings the things into the home for us. The community looks after us. It's all fine. We don't really need much. It's amazing what you can do without money, really.

KL: Well, it certainly sounds like you've done a lot of good there.

LJ: I enjoy sharing my knowledge with the children and seeing them grow and be happy.

KL: So, what happens next?

LJ: There's going to be a war.

KL: Oh! Who's the war between?

LJ: It's between England and Germany. The Germans are everywhere, and they are invading England, and we need to go and help them.

KL: What year is it?

LJ: It's 1942, but I think I'm too old to go, but I might have to.

KL: How old are you now? Do you remember what year you were born?

LJ: I guess I must be in my 40s, somewhere around there. Mm-hmm, I'm probably too old to go. I should go and put my name down. I don't really want to, but I feel I should go and help if I can.

KL: What happens next?

(Life Between Lives: Client now moves into another life between life. Where she meets the council to review her life and options moving forward).

LJ: I don't know what's happened. I'm back in the tunnel. I'm going through the tunnel.

KL: What are you doing in the tunnel?

LJ: Waiting.

KL: Do you have a body?

LJ: Sort of.

KL: What happened to your body? Look back and see what happened to your body.

LJ: It's just in pieces. I was clearing landmines. I was there one moment, and then I wasn't.

KL: Where were the landmines?

LJ: On the beach.

KL: Which country are you in?

LJ: I'm in France; I'm on the beach in France. I was trying to make the place safe for people to be able to go back to the beach.

KL: Did you get blown up?

LJ: Yeah.

KL: So, one minute you were there, the next you were back in the tunnel. So, what happens next?

LJ: I must wait my turn to review my contract. I've been here before. Maybe I'll choose a different door.

KL: What do they say?

LJ: I'm waiting a long time?

KL: Why is that? What can you see?

LJ: It's a bit like being in a cocoon, really, you can see a light at the end where the council are, but I just want to sleep here for a while. Like I must gather all the bits together.

KL: Let's condense time and move forward and see what happens next. What do you choose next?

LJ: I'm going to choose to have time out. We don't have to do anything straight away, and they are saying you can, if you want, go in and help someone else with their contract. You don't have to have a new contract yourself. You could just be like, you could just go play if you want, but you just promise you're going to help that person do one thing or two things to help them in their life.

KL: How does that work? Would you have a body or...

LJ: Not always. You don't have to have a body to do that. You can do that without a body; you could be just like a spirit entity that works with them.

KL: So, you could be like a guide, maybe supporting them?

LJ: Yeah. So, you don't have to have a physical body. So that sounds like quite a nice thing to do because if you do that, you get to go between different planes, and you don't just stay on the earth plane. And you can go, and you can bring more stuff from elsewhere, more information, whatever they're ready to receive, you collect that and bring it to them.

KL: So, what do you choose since you can choose whatever you like? Let's move forward and see what you choose.

LJ: Oh, apparently, you can go through the door and do that as well because you don't have to do that all the time. And you can do it for other people, not just one person. You can work with lots of people as a spirit entity, spirit guide, and you get to play all over again.

KL: So many choices; it sounds like fun.

LJ: You can get information from everywhere.

KL: You like your information. What are you going to choose then?

LJ: I'm going to be a guide; it sounds more fun than anything. Well, I think the hard part is getting people to listen to you. That's the tricky bit. That's a challenge. But it will be alright. There are quite a few people who do this.

KL: Are there people that you know? Do you recognise their energy?

LJ: No, it's not like people. Most people who are doing this are just having a great time. You might get a promotion (laughs). You're not to be naughty, though.

KL: Oh. So, what happens next?

LJ: You take on this role.

KL: Where do you go? What do you do?

LJ: Well, first, you get assigned to various people. Then they get a feeling and can see or hear you better. Sometimes, they just don't understand what you're telling them, which can be a bit frustrating. But when you get the message across, that's good. Sometimes they ask you things, and you must get the information so that they understand.

KL: I can imagine.

LJ: But then you get some good ones.

KL: So, do you have any good ones that you can connect with easily that listen?

LJ: Yeah, but they don't always listen when you want to tell them stuff. They listen when they want to listen. Mm-hmm. But when you get the message across to them, sometimes, they ask you things, and then you've got to go and find the answers. And they understand that it's challenging, but it's great because you can get some good stuff.

KL: What kind of good stuff?

LJ: I can show them what their path can be or what alternatives are open to them. Also, I can remind them of their contracts. And sometimes I can help put other people in their way—people who contract to do stuff with them together. Then, when they realise, they get that feeling. You know, when there's that connection, there's that buzzy fuzzy feeling that they get as well.

KL: You like it when that happens?

LJ: Yes, well, we can travel anywhere.

KL: Where do you travel to?

LJ: I go anywhere. And the earth is the most interesting.

KL: Oh, what's very interesting about diverse millions of people.

LJ: Sometimes, when you're visiting, if one of the people you are supposed to work with don't connect to you, you can be assigned to somebody else. You may just find that somebody else can sense or listen to you or hear you and then you may be allowed to connect with them.

KL: So, what type of people do you like time travel? Is there a particular interest or topic?

LJ: I don't think I have anything specific regarding that; I just love having that connection. It's just sometimes the most amazing feeling. When you get that connection, there's nothing quite like it, and for me, that's what it's all about—just having that moment. It's helping them. Sometimes, it's just almost being a comfort to them as well. You know, sometimes people are very sad, and they can feel someone else is there when there isn't anybody else there for them.

KL: That's nice. So, should we move forward and see what happens?

LJ: There's a chance to go on a time travel. You'd have to go in like a rocket when you think it'll be like uncapped; you know, it's interesting. For me, I want to know who else is going because now, they're showing me the rocket, and it only looks like there's room for one. Okay, so they're saying other people have done it, and they're in different time zones, different timelines. And if you choose a timeline, you will hook up with other people who have travelled on that timeline as well. So, there's like a whole raft of different realities—like a big network. You can just go along one line, and then sometimes you can jump. They're showing me a big image of how it works. There are all these lines going out, and if you don't want one of the lines, you can then jump to another reality, a different line at certain points. If you go on one, you don't have to stay on that one. So, if you don't like it, you can switch. But only at certain points. You can't just switch. You must wait for the opportunity to switch. It's like a switching point and until you get to that point, you can't switch; else, you just drop off.

KL: So, what do you choose?

LJ: We could do that, especially if I'm not going to be all on my own.

KL: Shall I do a drumroll? What are you going to choose?

LJ: Okay, so that's another way of doing it. You start off with all the points joined, and you can go along for a while, then you can make your choice, so you get to choose which timeline you want to go on.

KL: You like your options, don't you? So, you can try it and then you can change it?

LJ: Yeah. You just must wait for a switching point to choose another one. So, there's also another option in there. I was hearing switch. It's like an emergency button, but you can't keep pressing that button.

KL: Are there rules then about how many times you can press the switch?

LJ: You get a sense or a vision of the parallel and then if you want to stay on the line, you're on, you can. If not, you can just switch over and switch back once you're on that one, then you're off on backtrack, but there are other switching down choices.

KL: It sounds a little bit like the London Underground.

LJ: (Laughing) I think I'd love to go on this journey.

KL: Let's move forward and see what happens. Let's move forward to when you've made your choice.

LJ: It's weird. It's a bit like being in a library, but it's a reference library, and you can take a book and open that book, and you're in there. So, if you open the book on planets and the stars, you're in the planets and the stars, and you move through them and around them. When you're done, you can shut that book and go into a whole other world. You could look at flowers or people or whatever you want. That's when the switch comes as well. You can close that book because it's all about experiences, and you can totally submerge yourself in those experiences. Be part of it. Not like with a body.

KL: Is there a particular book that draws you into this library?

LJ: I think I could start with planets; you can go on for miles and miles, you might not come back. It is very beautiful. I might become a star myself, a shooting star, moving around the universe.

Reflections

At this point, the client came quickly out of the trance as they needed the bathroom. So, after her bathroom visit, we integrated all that had taken place. The client was surprised at the level of information that came through and the intensity of the feelings, saying that they felt so real. She had previously had a past life regression with another therapist some years ago but had got very vague information, so she said it was great to be able to go deeper this time and really get a feel for the day-to-day experience and the past life personality and character. The client has many similar character traits as the past life personality and had for the past few months volunteered as the events manager for her local church community. This was an interesting session as the client spent a lot of time in the life between lives section, I invited her several times to see if she wanted to move forward but she continued to explore the options. The client's higher self and guides are always guiding the session, so I'm sure this was important not only for the client but also for the project and for those who are or will be reading this book. I love that her higher self chose to present the many possibilities, choices, and timelines, and how we can and do jump tracks.

Akhenaten, Nefertiti, The Handmaiden & Tutankhamun

In this session, I connected my client with her higher self and invited her higher self to take her wherever she needed to go at this time. We ended up in a 'past life' in Egypt, with connections to Star-beings, and a rather interesting storyline.

ST: Ekashay.

KL: Ekashay? Hello.

ST: I'm seeing the pyramids in Egypt. I've come to reconnect with my soul group.

KL: Beautiful.

ST: Akhenaten, Nefertiti we are one of a kind, there is a mutual understanding with no judgement. I was close to them in court.

KL: What was your role in the court?

ST: I was a handmaiden. But I think that's what I've been told. But I believe I was a bit more than a handmaiden. I performed rituals in the pyramids.

KL: So just allow yourself to relax and go deeper and deeper and deeper into that memory, that time, space, place. Allow yourself to see clearly so that you can know for yourself, who you truly are.

ST: I'm seeing myself in one of the pyramids. It's a huge vast open space and I'm sitting with what I believe is a singing bowl, it's a huge black bowl. This is part of the ritual. I don't believe there are many people here, it's a very, very small audience and you for those who would understand.

KL: So, who else is there with you?

ST: Akhenaten, Nefertiti, and a few others. It's a private gathering.

KL: What's the ritual for?

ST: To reconnect, to call in our brothers and sisters, to have a sense of being there, being home. We weren't from this world we came down to create change.

KL: Can you tell us where you came from?

ST: I can hear the Pleiades but then Sirius. Again, I don't feel there's one place. We came down to connect. We came together. As in whilst we were here, we were drawn together.

KL: What do you mean drawn together?

ST: So, we didn't arrive together, we were in separate locations, but our energy was like a magnet, so we came together because that was the mission, that was the purpose.

KL: For what purpose did you come together?

ST: We came together to assist, create change, to assist in the evolution, to bring balance, consistency, calm to the lands, the sacred lands.

KL: Did you come to just one place in Egypt or were there other locations that you came to on earth?

ST: I don't understand the question.

KL: When you came to the earth did you come into just one location, or did you come to many locations?

ST: Our main objective was to be in Egypt, in that area. We also generated an extreme amount of energy and power. We assisted and enabled the energy to come through into the lands. That was also part of the mission to clear the lands.

KL: And what were you clearing from the land?

ST: The accumulation of humanity's negativity that had been absorbed into the sacred land. We assisted to bring through a higher frequency, lighter energy, to be able to flow through the sacred land. I'm now seeing from the pyramids, beams of light coming out from the points, these reach high up into the sky into the out through the atmosphere of the earth.

KL: Can you say some more about the beams of light?

ST: The beams of light, yes. This is like a landmark, it's an energy portal that is seen easily from space. They go deep, deep into the earth, they're not seen by those who do not have a certain level of consciousness. Most normal people would not see this. When we go into the pyramids, we perform what you would call our rituals, we reconnect with this light. It enables us to communicate. We energise and heal the energy bodies of density.

KL: And is there anything else that you wish to tell us today or are there other beings, other aspects that want to come forward?

ST: I wish to tell you about the demise of the kingdom.

KL: Please continue.

ST: The peoples of the land were... I want to say poisoned, but that's the wrong word. They were brainwashed, and our status was not as favourable as it had been in the past. There were many in power, who were powerful leaders who were not happy with the way that we conducted our rituals they were not happy with who we were. There was an enormous amount of judgement towards us.

KL: And would we know any of those people in history? Are there any particular people or beings that were responsible for the brainwashing?

ST: They were your, what you would call priests. Respected men, that were respected by many and that's why it was easy for them to portray a negative image.

KL: Were some of these priests also kings or rulers or pharaohs?

ST: They were in line for the throne. Their motif was for their own gratification. Whispers in corridors, you know this happens frequently through the ages, there is so much corruption within royalty, they are very good at influencing. I have experienced this in many lifetimes, being within court I am fully aware of how to conduct myself in court. How to Survive.

KL: Were you yourself in the royal lineage?

ST: I was not royalty myself in this lifetime. I was assisting Akhenaten, and Nefertiti. I was within the court, but I was not one of royalty.

KL: Are Akhenaten and Nefertiti with you now?

ST: I feel Akhenaten often comes into my energy field to assist and help me. Nefertiti more so in the early days, but she occasionally pops in. I feel their essence is here, but I do not believe they are here at this precise moment. I feel that I had a child in this lifetime. There was secrecy about the father of that child.

KL: Who was the father of the child?

ST: I'm slightly confused by who that is. But I'm sensing that I had a child, but I don't know who with, it was with somebody in the court.

KL: I see, did you have a boy or girl?

ST: A boy.

KL: What did you name him?

ST: Oh! (Client crying) I know who he was. Tutankhamun! Such corruption.

KL: So, you said that it was a secret? (Yes) Why did it need to be a secret?

ST: Because I was just purely a handmaiden, and the father was King.

KL: What happens to your son?

ST: He was next in line to the throne.

KL: And what did the king's wife think about that?

ST: I do not feel that she was upset by it. I'm sensing that there needed to be this child. Because I was of the human form. Nefertiti and Akhenaten were not of the human form and because of the judgement and the resistance that was experienced the bloodline needs to be diluted.

KL: And so, what happens after the birth of your child?

ST: I was hidden for the duration of pregnancy, and I gave birth and had to give him away.

KL: Who looked after him?

ST: I was part of the team that looked after him. I was his wet nurse. I still played a role as mother, although one of secrecy. I'm not sure what I'm seeing but I'm not sure if Nefertiti is the mother. I feel there is another wife. A quiet and timid woman.

KL: Have you seen her before?

ST: She is within the court. She is not part of Akhenaten and Nefertiti's lineage. She is of royal lineage by birth.

KL: Hmm. Can you describe her?

ST: She's small, fairly young.

KL: What kind of hair has she got?

ST: She has black hair. She is very beautiful. She's nearly a child herself.

KL: Is she a good mother figure?

ST: You must remember that when you compare a mother to how a mother is now to mother, back then it was very, very different. It was merely a status symbol. You had many people assisting in the process of bringing up that child. I don't... there was no real love. There's quite an empty relationship between the two. But obviously, she did not have that physical bond with that child.

KL: Did you stay close to your son?

ST: Yes, I was part of the court. I was his wet nurse, and I assisted in his upbringing.

KL: And for how long were you able to stay close to him? Were you always close?

ST: Yes. This has happened in other lifetimes.

KL: Did you share your knowledge and rituals with your son?

ST: I did not he was unaware of his real mother.

KL: Did you continue to do ceremonies for the court?

ST: I believe I did not. Tension was beginning. The tension was growing. It was not advisable at that time to be doing our prayer and ritual.

KL: So, let's move forward. Let's condense time and move forward to the next significant time.

ST: Akhenaten has been murdered with a dagger to the heart.

KL: Who would do such a thing?

ST: You must remember the corruption in court.

KL: Do you know who did this?

ST: It was a female.

KL: Do you know who the female was? Was she family to Akhenaten?

ST: Not directly. There's some confusion as to who's done it.

KL: How do you know that it was a female?

ST: That is a very good question. She had no choice.

KL: Why was it that she had no choice. Your secret's safe with us.

ST: Because she had to protect the future King.

KL: So, she was protecting Tutankhamun and was she connected with Tutankhamun?

ST: Yes. She was indirectly connected.

KL: Indirectly connected in what way? Are you able to tell me?

ST: Sometimes great sacrifice needs to be experienced for the benefit of others. When you look at the bigger picture and when you look into the future of the people, of the land. We need to consider every option. Some decisions that we undertake are for the benefit of others.

KL: Perhaps this is something that we can come back to we don't have too much longer left right now. Sonya needs to be somewhere.

ST: Yes.

KL: Is there anything else that you wish to say before you leave?

ST: Only that the soul is limitless. There are infinite opportunities in the future and never to never to take your current experience as something that is going to continue forever. Life is like an ocean. The waves, the water coming into shore is endless. It's an endless cycle of ebbs and flows the soul is very much the same as that sea. It is endless, limitless

KL: Thank you very much for speaking with us today Thank you. Perhaps we'll see you again. Yes. So, Sonya, just taking a nice deep, relaxing breath and just allowing any beings to step back. bringing forward the wisdom, the knowledge, the connections, the memory, perhaps those gifts and abilities that you can integrate into this lifetime. Knowing that you're always guided just bringing yourself back into full waking consciousness. Allowing that white light to bring you back to your body back into this 3d physical reality becoming aware of your feet on the floor. Aware of your physical body very gently when you're ready opening your eyes, coming back feeling refreshed, wide awake, remembering all that you need to remember and leaving anything that no longer serves behind.

Debrief with the Client.

ST: Oh, that was a bit heavy going, but it all makes sense now because when I used to go into trance Tutankhamun used to come through a lot. I've always known that there was this link between the three of them and myself. I knew that I was a handmaiden to Nefertiti but it's interesting how the lifetimes can repeat themselves. Because I've had exactly the same life in another time.

KL: Being a handmaiden do you mean?

ST: Being within the court. The presence within the court and having a child again um yeah, that's interesting.

ST: What did you sense? Who do you think killed him?

KL: I don't know. I'm curious. Maybe we'll find out some more.

ST: Yes. I know.

KL: You know. (Yeah.) Who was it then?

ST: I just don't want to say.

KL: Why not?

ST: Because.

KL: Why?

ST: I don't know.

KL: Did you, do it?

ST: Yeah.

KL: I thought that. (When I say I thought that, what I mean is that I was aware that the client thought she as the handmaiden and true mother to Tutankhamun had done it.

ST: And it's interesting because I've seen that vision before. I don't feel there's any malice. He understood. He knew what was going on. I know, because of who he was. He understood the bigger picture that the gain was huge compared to the loss. But it's interesting how I saw the Egyptian with you. I think that was like the calling card. You're going to Egypt. Oh, yeah. I was waiting on the Egypt one to come out I thought when is the Egypt one going to come out?

ST: Could I make this up? I don't know perhaps that's just me thinking well, how could little old me be…Do you know what I mean?

KL: Well, it's possible, but why would you?

ST: I don't know, it's just it seems unbelievable. Does that make sense?

KL: You know, let's talk about it some other time when you're not going. During this session, the number 44 1440 1144 144. Fours are all to do with balance, family, and foundation, platform. It's also of course the 144,000.

Reflections

So, did the client really give birth to Tutankhamun? Maybe, maybe not. This could be a result of imprinting or mediumship and following the session, I did speak with the client about the possibilities. It is, however, an interesting story and of course, the connection with royalty, being in court has come up a couple of times with this client. I can see how valuable it would be for the client to connect more fully with her power and sovereignty in order to step more fully into her role as a leader and to get her gifts out into the world. I always invite the client's higher self, to download the lessons, blessings and gifts and I trust that the client's higher self will show them what's required for their greater understanding and will support the client in integrating all that unfolds within the session. Sometimes further integration and insight comes in meditation, or in dreams, or journaling, channelling or subsequent connection or sessions with the higher self.

The American Civil War & The Lords of Light

This client is a healer and channel and has been exploring issues around visibility, personal leadership, and sovereignty. She starts off in a past life and then we move into life between lives, where she meets the Lords of Light before going into another past life.

ST: I'm in the Amazon jungle. It's a journey I often go on. So, I've got into a dug-out boat that takes me along the river until we meet a waterfall. I get out of the boat and walk under the waterfall into a cave—a crystal cave. I imagine myself on this chair in the cave.

KL: Okay, so as you're sitting on this chair, look around and see what crystals are there.

ST: Oh, it's very glistening. The word coming to mind is selenite, some clear quartz, some deep sort of royal blue flecks of gold.

KL: Beautiful. Yeah. So just allow yourself to relax in this beautiful crystal cave and allow the energies of the crystals to take you deeper and deeper. Just letting go, allowing yourself to drift, simply being, sensing, allowing the crystals to contribute to you, to your body, to your being. Allow yourself to relax deeper and deeper so that you can begin to be aware of energies, any beings with bodies or without bodies, those aspects of yourself that we might call multi-dimensional.

ST: I keep seeing this picture, and it's not very pleasant.

The client is clearing her throat a lot.

KL: Okay.

ST: I'm a male. And it's not pleasant. Somebody has forked me in the neck. And I'm stuck.

KL: Okay, is that what's going on with your throat?

ST: Maybe. Yeah. They've pierced me in the neck, and I'm stuck.

KL: Okay. Where are you?

ST: I feel I'm on a battlefield.

KL: Okay. And do you want to rewind and see a little bit of context? Have a look and see what you're wearing?

ST: I've got the word Roman coming to mind.

KL: Okay, so have a look down at your feet, your body and see what you're wearing.

ST: I've got black boots and I'm wearing tight jodhpur trousers.

KL: Okay.

ST: And the jacket has gold buttons. I think it's white. White with red.

KL: How old are you?

ST: Not young; sort of 30s. Something like that.

KL: What are you doing on this battlefield?

ST: I think I'm part of the battle.

KL: Who are you fighting? Which country are you from? Where are you?

ST: I'm not sure; I do not see who they are.

KL: Okay. Are there any other people there with you?

ST: There are, but I can't see them. I just know that they're there. It's like, I've sort of feel a bit like I'm on my own, but I'm not.

KL: Okay. So, are you in your body? Are you out of your body?

ST: I think I'm in my body because I feel trapped by this fork in my neck.

KL: Aha. Can you see the face of the person who's got the hole in your neck?

ST: No, no. No.

KL: Okay, so what happens next?

ST: I'm just lying there, trapped with this fork in my neck.

KL: So, are you dead?

ST: I don't believe I am dead. Not yet.

KL: Okay. So, do you want to fast forward or rewind? Imagine it's like a movie.

ST: I think I just need to accept that perhaps that's maybe a past life.

KL: Take some nice deep breaths. Allow yourself to relax. And you can be aware of the fork in it. And just know that you can experience this without any discomfort. Yes, you can be here and there. And your unconscious mind has brought this in for a reason. Let's explore and see what's happening. Okay, what's the relevance? So, you can rewind and get some more detail in terms of who you are, what country you're from, where you are, where you're fighting. Or you can fast forward, and we can kind of see what happens.

ST: Yeah, I'm kind of seeing more now. I see cannons, black cannons. Okay. I'm not sure, but I think that I'm American. Maybe this is the Civil War. I'm not sure. I feel that I'm American or something like that. There's many of us. I feel this war has been going on for a long time. We're all quite tired. It seems to never end.

KL: So, do you have family in this lifetime?

ST: I don't know.

KL: Let's fast forward and see what happens as you move forward.

ST: Okay, yeah, I'm now back home. I'm at my home. I don't know if it's after the war, but I think I'm like a farmer with my family on the farm. I believe this is America. I have a wife and children, and we have a farm. It's a simple life.

KL: Ah so you escaped from the fork in your neck and you're on the farm with your family—wife, and children.

ST: Yeah.

KL: How old are you?

ST: I don't know. I'm not sure.

KL: How old are your children? Can you see them?

ST: They're quite young.

KL: How many children do you have?

ST: Two children. One girl, one boy. I think they're eight.

KL: So, one's eight? The girl or the boy?

ST: The boy.

KL: And the daughter?

ST: She's roughly about the same age. Ten or something like that. I'm not sure.

KL: What's your name?

ST: Jacob.

KL: What's your wife's name?

ST: Marion.

KL: Marion. Okay. So, what happens in this life? Let's move forward to the next significant event.

ST: Ah, I see Quakers.

KL: Okay. And are you a Quaker?

ST: I believe so.

KL: What's happening now, Jacob?

ST: I'm just seeing all the Quaker people on their horse and carts and just going about their business.

KL: Are you seeing this like a movie?

ST: I'm kind of seeing it through his eyes.

KL: Yeah. So just take a nice deep breath. As you breathe out, slip into that picture so that you can become Jacob, allowing yourself to go deeper and deeper, more and more relaxed. Getting a sense of your body.

ST: I feel like we were a really happy community, quite separate from the others. We kept to ourselves. But they kept interfering with us with the way that we lived our lives and the way that we wanted to live.

KL: They kept interfering?

ST: The authorities, okay, those that were in power.

KL: In what way do they interfere?

ST: Oh, coming in, telling us what to do, how to do things, and trying to get us to comply with their rules. We were quite happy just being the way that we were. I think they were the ones that made me go to war. I didn't want to fight but I had no choice.

KL: To fight?

ST: Yes, I felt quite helpless. Oh, oh. I think they came into the community. And they burnt all the houses down. They didn't like us. They wanted to get rid of us. Because we were different from them, so they burned all our homes. They try to push us out.

KL: Did they push you out?

ST: Yes. We had to move on. We very gradually created another settlement. I feel that the brutality continued. It didn't stop. Wherever we went, they would come and try and interfere and get us to try and live in a way that we weren't happy with living.

KL: How did that impact you and your family and community?

ST: We felt very trapped. We couldn't relax. We always felt on edge. Because we never know when they would come into the village. Yeah. They always came in with many of them; there was always force.

KL: Let's move forward. So just fast forward to the next significant time in this lifetime.

ST: I feel I'm now old. They did eventually leave us alone. We did continue to create our settlement. The authorities oversaw us from a distance. They had less interaction with our system. I went on, but I feel I'm old now. I want to say eighty-seven. I feel quite settled; I feel I'm coming to the end of my life

KL: What makes you think that?

ST: Because I feel a sense of completion, it's time to move on.

KL: How is your body physically?

ST: There's no injury or anything. It's just natural. The body's aged.

KL: What happens next?

ST: I'm lying in my bed with my family around me. I think I'm moving on. I think it's now time to move on. To leave this world, I feel a little anxious about that.

KL: What do you feel anxious about?

ST: Well because I'm leaving my family. Yeah. I feel a little sad about that, but... Oh, I see the bright light and singing. It's very peaceful.

The client is moving into a life between lives.

KL*: Are you in your body, or have you left your body now?*

ST: I've left my body now. I feel like I'm with two beings.

KL*: Do you know those two beings?*

ST: Yes.

KL: *Do you know their names?*

ST: I'm not sure. I don't know how to say their name. They feel familiar, but I'm not sure.

KL: Do you see their faces?

ST: I don't see their faces yet. But they are wearing white cloaks and they have gold headdresses.

KL: Are they male or female?

ST: I don't feel they have a gender. One is the energy of blue, and the other is the energy of red.

KL: What do they feel like? What's their energy like?

ST: They feel loving, like mother and father. They feel welcoming.

KL: Do they find anything to talk to you about?

ST: They're just standing there, waiting.

KL: What are they waiting for?

ST: I think they're waiting for me to come closer. I think they're here to welcome me back.

KL: Do you want to move closer to them?

ST: Yes. I'm sensing the words, Lords of Light.

KL: Lords of Light? Okay.

ST: They are familiar, and I see these big gates, huge, ornately carved gates, white gates. I feel they are the Lords of Light. I now can see their faces. They are not human. They are humanoid. But their faces are not human. They are very sculptured. Their cheekbones are very sculptured, not like our cheekbones.

KL: What is the colour of their skin?

ST: They have like a whitish shimmering, luminous see-through skin, small eyes, peculiar mouth, and nose.

KL: In what way peculiar?

ST: Well, peculiar because if I was comparing them to a human, they are nothing like a human at all

KL: Do you feel comfortable with them?

ST: Yes.

KL: So, what happens next?

ST: They are inviting me in through the doors—these big gates. They do not speak. I understand them. I can see that the doors, the gates, whatever you want to call them, are opening very slowly. Through mind control. It's like our minds are controlling these gates; they open very slowly. It feels like all three of our minds when we are all ready. Yeah, we feel like we are all ready to walk through these gates. They very slowly open.

KL: So, are they communicating with you telepathically?

ST: Yes, I believe so.

KL: Or is it just a feeling?

ST: Well, it's a feeling, but I believe this is telepathy. So, as we walk through these gates, everything becomes really bright as though I'm perhaps somewhere different, but not different. It's hard to explain, just this really bright, welcoming light.

KL: Oh!

ST: I can see many other beings waiting there. They've been waiting for me.

KL: Are these beings familiar to you?

ST: Yes, but there are many. There are so many different diverse beings they're not all the same. They are very different.

KL: Can you describe some of them?

ST: I don't know where to begin.

KL: Is there anybody you recognise?

ST: There aren't any humans here. They're all humanoid. Their structures are all very different. Some are tall, some thin, some long. Some of the humanoids wear clothes, and some don't wear clothes. Some have big heads. Some have small heads; some have small eyes, some big eyes. There is such variation. Some are what you would classify as animal like yeah, they feel very familiar.

KL: And where do you feel you are?

ST: I feel like I'm a void of space. I can't tell you where I am. It doesn't feel like I'm anywhere, but I'm in this void, this space.

KL: Can you ask the Lords of Light where this space is?

ST: Another dimension. I feel I'm part of this group.

KL: Wonderful.

ST: Yes, I feel that I have done this many times. Gone to earth and come back.

KL: So, are you on the planet? Are you in heaven?

ST: I suppose if I was to give it words, heaven would be a more understandable way of describing it. But I would call it the void—the void in time and space.

KL: How do you feel?

ST: I don't feel that I'm going to be here for long.

KL: Okay. Let's move forward to the next significant time.

The client now moves into another life.

ST: I'm sensing a baby; I feel I have taken shape and form. I've come back to the physical earth plane to experience and have a better understanding.

KL: What is it that you're here to have a better understanding of?

ST: What it's like to be in a physical body, and what it is like to be here. We wish to understand what it is like to be here in this physical place.

KL: Is there a particular mission that you've come in with the purpose of this lifetime?

ST: We always come with the best intention to learn, to try and bring some peace, some love. We try to show people that there's a better way to be and a better way of being. That war is not necessary. I feel that life before was necessary for me to experience what war is. Now I feel that I'm being born into the end of the war. I'm being born into a time of peace, a time of growth—expansion where humanity feels senses with the heart than they do with the mind.

KL: What country are you in?

ST: America, I believe.

KL: And can you see your parents?

ST: Basically, yes. They look a bit hippie. Uh-huh. Well, we would call them hippies.

KL: Do you have a name?

ST: I don't know.

KL: What do your parents call you?

ST: I'm not sure.

KL: Ok, so just take a moment to get a sense of your body and how old you are.

ST: I'm a baby. Yeah. I've just been born.

KL: Ah, you've just been born. Okay. So where are you?

ST: I'm still in the hospital. They're admiring me. They love their new baby; their hearts are filled with joy. They do not realise that I can sense that. That I'm so much more than a baby, a human baby. It's a very happy place. There's lots of love. I feel there's a lot of love in this part of the hospital. It's very happy.

KL: Are you male or female?

ST: I'm female.

KL: So, you're a beautiful baby girl.

ST: Yes.

KL: Would you like to move forward? See what happens in this lifetime?

ST: Yes.

KL: Just fast forward to a significant time in this life.

ST: Yes. It is a time of peace. A time of movement; people came together to create peace. I feel I'm part of that movement. I feel that that's why I'm here. I see lots of people on the streets protesting very peacefully for peace.

KL: And how old are you now?

ST: I feel I'm in my early 20s.

KL: Where in America are you living?

ST: In Washington, I think.

KL: Do you know who the president is.

ST: I can see him, but I can't think of his name. I think he got shot. I'm not sure. I have a feeling that I don't live very long in this body. I'm taken with cancer; it was a very, very short life.

KL: Are you single? Do you have a family?

ST: I have a young family. I have one child or a young child. It was very sad, quite tragic. I can't quite tell, but my time has come to move on. I have done what I came here to do, and it's now time to move on. I'm sensing that with every incarnation, the mission is getting closer to the end goal. Does that make sense in any way to you?

KL: So, what is the end goal?

ST: The end goal is now.

KL: So, what is your mission in this lifetime?

ST: To awaken, to be a beacon of light, to bring about truths, unity. We're getting closer, closer to when humanity is ready to make contact with what you would classify as the unseen world; it's always been present. Humanity has been unable to perceive, partly because they are unable and partly to do with the way that they live their lives.

KL: So, when we say the unseen world, are you referring to the spirit world? Are you referring to different types of beings?

ST: I am referring to the worlds beyond earth. The majority of the human population are unable to perceive this, but there are many who do perceive it.

KL: So, your role is to enable more of humanity to perceive these other realms, worlds.

ST: Yes, to prepare them.

KL: And what are you preparing them for?

ST: Integration with the unseen world.

KL: So, where are you now?

ST: I feel there's a big discussion going on. I feel it has to do with what to do next.

KL: Are you there in the discussion?

ST: On the fringes.

KL: Who's having the discussion?

ST: I'm trying to put it into words you would understand.

KL: Can you see these people?

ST: Yes, they are very advanced. I want to say superior, but that's not in any way; they're not in charge of anybody or authority over anybody. They are evolved beings.

KL: And this is their role in helping people choose?

ST: Their role is to oversee the evolution of humanity and the integration process.

KL: So, they're helping souls on the journey.

ST: Yes. How best can we serve, for that is what we wish to do. We wish to be part of this great expansion.

KL: When you say we, who do you mean?

ST: All of the beings wish to contribute in a positive and meaningful manner. We all wish to serve and to spread our light now?

KL: What are they discussing about your life? What's next your mission?

ST: How best to integrate me into society? How my life will develop and what I will do for this life they are discussing feels in comparison to the other life that I've had. It feels like it has more purpose. It feels like I'm getting closer to really delivering what is needed, what is required. I feel the other lives have been very much about trying to understand the life on this earth.

KL: So, they've been preparing you for those lifetimes?

ST: Yes, this feels very much like I will be able to be more myself in my soul body, as opposed to being in a body of learning. I will be in a body where I'm able to emit my own light, to express my own light in a way that is more familiar to me. As opposed to being more familiar with those that I'm with.

KL: Yeah. So, what happens next?

ST: I feel I'm going to be born in 1970, which is the body that I'm in now; that's what it feels like.

KL: How many lives have you heard on earth in total prior to this?

ST: Many. Hundreds and hundreds.

KL: Have they always been on earth?

ST: No, I have chosen to come down at particular points in time to experience the development at that time. It is not like I have come down, been born, did that life, died, gone up, come back straightaway. I have been born on the earth plane at pivotal points in time. So, although I say perhaps hundreds of lives on the earth plane, they have been over many, many years. Hundreds of thousands of years.

KL: So, is there anything in this lifetime, any experiences or times in this lifetime that are significant for you to see that your unconscious wants you to see?

ST: There have been times of quiet contemplation where I have been creating a pathway that is favourable for me to complete my mission. My mother plays a very big part in this mission. She is a light-bearer; she is able to be grounded in the light to enable high vibrational frequencies to be powered within the body. You could say she's like a battery. She will continue that role throughout the physical body that she's in now and when she passes over. For example, if I was to be born into a different family where my mother was not the way she is, I would not be able to incorporate the amount of light that I have been able to on this earth.

KL: Have you been with your mother before in other lifetimes?

ST: Yes.

KL: So, you made a good choice.

ST: Yes. It's all planned.

KL: And how about your father?

ST: My dear father, with the greatest respect in every way, was the vehicle to create my existence.

KL: What gifts have you received from your father?

ST: Mainly earthly gifts. How to best live life here; life skills.

KL: Well, those are important, right?

ST: Yes, very much; it helps in the transition. What I mean by that are the experiences that you will have throughout your life, if you make the right choices, because of your experience, and it will create a smoother transitional period of life.

KL: So, you mean a smoother journey in life?

ST: A smoother journey in this physical body.

KL: Have you travelled with your father before in this lifetime?

ST: No, I do not believe so.

KL: Okay. So, is there anything else that you need from this lifetime? Or do you want to come back, or do you want to go somewhere else?

ST: All is well.

KL: Can I just check in with your higher self and with your body to see if there's anything that needs to be resolved from that life with the pitchfork in your neck?

ST: The soul. The benevolent, loving soul struggles somewhat with conflicts and war. That lifetime was to have a better understanding of that.

KL: So, what did she actually learn from that? What did she come to understand?

ST: I learned physical pain—pain through loss and helplessness. I saw the darker side of what it means to be here.

KL: And what did you learn from those experiences?

ST: I learned a lot about the vibration that they hold and how a whole race of people can be guided from that lower energy. The next life was very much about the opposite of that.

KL: So, you're talking about the collective consciousness and its impacts?

ST: Yes. Yes.

KL: Very powerful learnings. So, I'm wondering, in this life, too, does she have any issues with her throat physically, or any issues around communication and conflict expressing herself?

ST: Yes, very much.

KL: I'm wondering whether we can clear all and any cellular memory from her throat and release those lessons that were learned in that lifetime regarding conflict and lower vibrations, the helplessness?

ST: Yes.

KL: Let's just ask Source and your higher self to heal and clear physically, mentally, emotionally, spiritually, anything that needs to be released from that lifetime and that you have all the lessons, the blessings, and the gifts, and you can let go of any sadness or sorrow or any fear, physical pain, loss, helplessness, and that you already have these lessons, that they are completed. And I'm wondering whether there were any beings or any karma from that life when you were in battle.

ST: I do not feel so.

KL: So that's all resolved. That's good. Okay, is there anything else that's required to integrate that lifetime? (No.) Okay. And from the other lifetime, when you died young with cancer, is there anything from that lifetime that's required to be resolved that you can integrate that? (No.) Okay. So, does your higher self have any message or guidance for you?

ST: I know this, but I'm being reminded, there is support. In times of challenge, struggle and when everything around me is falling apart, I will always have my spiritual connection. There will be that immense light surrounding me, infusing me. I need to remember that there are many beings who are with me, guiding me, supporting me in the journey.

KL: That's always good to know. I wonder if there are any parts of you in this life that are required to be integrated or perhaps not aware of that light?

ST: There has been much integration in recent years. There is still much light to be put into the body, and over the next few years, this integration process will increase as we get closer to what we would classify as the pivotal point, the purpose of life.

KL: When will that pivotal point be in earth times?

ST: In the later years, in her 50s and into the 60s.

KL: At that point, what will happen?

ST: She will have fully embodied the light; there will be 100% light integration.

KL: Beautiful, and then what will happen?

ST: She will be a very different person.

Reflections

This was another wonderful session where the client was able to connect with a lifetime that was linked with an injury to her throat and neck to then heal and release unconscious beliefs and feelings, memories that were keeping her from being visible and speaking out. The client has had issues in this life with speaking out and problems in her earlier life speaking as she had a stutter.

I feel the client's higher self and guides were aware of the purpose of this project and wanting to come forward to share information as well as to strengthen the connections and give the client more opportunity to channel.

In this session, my client was wanting to connect more with her gifts and abilities. She has a lot of abilities and she's not showing up sharing them as she wants to. I invited her higher self to take her to whatever she needed to see and experience.

ST: I believe I'm in a place in Peru. I think it's called Touka or something like that.

KL: What are you doing there?

ST: I live there with my tribe.

KL: So just take a moment to look down at your feet and tell me what you have on your feet.

ST: Nothing. My feet are bare.

KL: And what else are you wearing?

ST: Very simple clothes made of reeds.

KL: Are you male or female?

ST: I'm male. I can tell by looking at my feet, they're so big.

KL: So, do you have a name?

ST: Tyrian.

KL: Okay. I'm not sure if I'm going to pronounce that properly.

ST: You can call me Terry.

KL: Terry. Okay, I can manage that. So, tell me about your life. Do you have a family?

ST: We are we are one big family. I don't believe I have a family as such now. But we are one big family.

KL: That's nice. Is that good to have one big family?

ST: Yes.

KL: How old are you?

ST: I'd say I'm in my prime? I want to say 30s. But between sort of, I don't know kind of 20-30s I'm quite young.

KL: So, you're in your prime. And how do you spend your daily life?

ST: So, we spend our daily lives going to the temples. And I in particular am in contact with what you call ET beings, Sky beings.

KL: And what's your role in that contact with the sky beings?

ST: I am an intermediate. So, I instigate communication with the sky beings.

KL: So how do you communicate with the sky beings?

ST: I have a big golden disc that I use. It is we place it at the top of the temple high up.

KL: Can you describe the temple?

ST: So, the temple is a very tall structure, with very many steps going up to a platform. We build them very tall so we can reach the sky people easier.

KL: Is it what we would call a stepped pyramid?

ST: Yes, similar, but there's no point at the top. It's flat.

KL: Why is it flat at the top?

ST: Because it's a platform.

KL: A platform for what?

ST: So, we can stand at this high point, it brings us closer to the sky people.

KL: Okay, so you said you have a golden disc?

ST: Yes, a bit like a gong. But it's not used as a gong or for that type of purpose. Generally, when the sun is at its highest point the sun reflects off the disc. This is the time that is more favourable to connect and contact. I want to say, gods.

KL: And these gods that you contact and connect with, where do they come from?

ST: They come from the stars.

KL: Is there a particular star that they come from or a particular group of stars?

ST: At the time, I was not aware of any particular star.

KL: Would Sonya know the stars?

ST: Yeah, Pleiades.

KL: Okay. so Tiri tell us about these star beings that you connected with, what kind of information or kind of connection do you have with them?

ST: When we look at the sky at night, we just see the sea of stars twinkling the moon, we see the sunrise and the moonrise, we ponder, and we wonder what's up there? And I felt the need to connect with something. I didn't know what I felt that there was more to what was within the night sky. I felt there was more to what was within the night. There was something out there. And the people were very interested, they wanted to explore this theory.

KL: Is that something that was taught, was that in the history of your family to watch the stars?

ST: Yes, they assisted us in the beginning, with planting cycles for crops. This relationship grew.

KL: Was that relationship with all the people, or do you have particular people that connect with the star beings?

ST: So, you have specific people like myself, who are the ones who connect with them, bring them through if you like. They are the intermediate. I can't say the word. You know what I mean.

KL: So, you're the intermediary? (Yes.) So, you connect with the star beings and then you relay their messages. (Yes.) What kinds of messages do they bring you?

ST: They bring us messages of hope. They sometimes assist us if, in times of struggle, they assist us, they raise our hope that there will be enough food. They bring us comfort.

KL: So, can we move forward in this lifetime and see what happens? Just taking a breath and allowing yourself to move to the next significant time.

ST: I'm now sensing the sky people have come here. Physically come here.

KL: So, do they come physically often?

ST: Not too often, periodically. They come in a ship.

KL: So, like a spaceship?

ST: Yeah. Like a disc, a bright light disc.

KL: Has it got a particular shape?

ST: I'm trying to think of the chocolate. It's got a hard shell. You get them in revels.

KL: Minstrels?

ST: Yeah, I think so is that them? They're not a disc. They're raised in the middle.

KL: Okay, so it's kind of like a disc shape that's raised in the middle. What do these beings look like? Can you see them?

ST: Yeah, they're quite different to us. They have very white pale skin, almost translucent. Their skin doesn't look like our skin at all. It's very different and their faces are very different. They have eyes, but they're bigger. And their bone structures are more carved, more pronounced. Their noses are smaller. Their mouths are smaller. They don't have ears.

KL: No ears?

ST: No ears. They have necks but they're long and thin. Their bodies are longer and thinner, smaller, longer arms. longer legs.

KL: What do they wear?

ST: They wear a long cloak. Very fancy, swishes and sways. It's made of very shimmering, glittery material like the stars, the way they shimmer. Their feet are similar, but they only have one big toe and a middle toe, and a small toe, and their feet are very wide near the toes. Imagine like my feet, but a lot wider at the end. So, they're very different to us. But they feel somewhat familiar to me. When I saw them, it felt very familiar? It didn't shock me. At first many of us were very scared, because we'd never seen these people before and in time, they grew to trust the relationship that we had. I taught them that these people come in peace they help us.

KL: You said they come physically now in the ship. What's the purpose of their visit?

ST: To make contact to create a bond to teach us better ways of doing things. teaching us about crop rotation and better ways to irrigate the land to produce more food. I'm sensing that there is mutual respect for the earth and the flow of the earth. They see how everything is interconnected and they teach us the importance of respecting the earth. I wonder if the other tribes in other places are in contact with these beings.

KL: The beings don't talk about that with you?

ST: No. I sense there are some teachings with regards to time, how to calculate time.

KL: It sounds as if they have a lot of wisdom.

ST: Oh yes, they come to teach us how to live better lives. I see my people celebrating. We get dressed up. We put paint on our faces, and we dance around the fire, calling and inviting the sky people to come and visit us if you like you could call it a ritual.

KL: Are you a shaman priest?

ST: If that is what you would wish to call me. Yes.

KL: Is that a part of your role?

ST: Yes. I am a healer as well. People come to me for healing

KL: What do you eat at the celebrations?

ST: We eat meat. Hog meat on the fire. I'm seeing a stone structure on either side and there is a thick piece of wood that goes over the top and the animal is put there, and it is turned periodically over the fire. I feel I must tell you about something else. I must tell you about the Crystal Skull.

KL: Oh, please do.

ST: There is a crystal skull in one of our temples. It was a gift from the sky people. We have it in a special temple on a stone plinth quite high up. This crystal skull is very powerful. When you touch the skull, you feel its wisdom. We can feel the stars, the moon, the sun. We can feel that space, that endless blackness. Only certain people are allowed to touch the skull.

KL: Are you're one of those people?

ST: Yeah. The skull is very dear to me. I feel it is a way of contacting the sky people without them being present the information that they would give us we can this information comes from the skull

KL: Beautiful, I'm wondering what type of skull it is?

ST: It's clear with some sort of markings in the middle it has cloudy bits. It's not completely clear. When you look inside you can see the moon and the stars glistening.

KL: Beautiful. So, shall we move forward in time?

ST: I feel I have caught a fever.

KL: Oh dear.

ST: There are people around me. They are placing special leaves upon my body to take the fever out of my body. I feel it's time to move on. Within our temples there are many carvings that tell the story of our progress. My time is done.

KL: What happens next?

ST: I feel I have left this body. We're united with those sky people, and it seems so much clearer now, more familiar. I understand now. I understand what that life was about.

KL: What were you learning from that life?

ST: My life was to enlighten, to bring hope, to reconnect with the sky people. To bring knowledge and to assist in the progression of the people. Famine was common. We needed assistance. For them to thrive they needed knowledge.

KL: So, you were the intermediary in that lifetime, bringing through knowledge. Were you pleased with that life and how it went?

ST: Yes.

KL: And so, what happens now?

ST: I feel they are discussing what is the best to do next? I feel these lords of light, they know what is best.

KL: These lords of light are they Pleiadean beings?

ST: They're Lyran.

KL: Can you describe them?

ST: They're the ones I described earlier. He has a big golden crown. They are the overseers, the watchers. They know what is best. They know there is always a choice. I do not wish to pursue their instructions, but it's okay because I do wish to be of assistance. So, it is an honour to take their instruction.

KL: So, they guide you into your next experience?

ST: Yes.

KL: Where are you going next?

ST: I'm feeling I'm moving continents now. I feel I'm going to the Americas. The Indian tribes are familiar to me. I know all these beings these tribal people are very familiar to me.

KL: What tribes are they?

ST: They are what you would call Native American Indians they assisted me greatly in this current life now.

KL: Are they tribes? Are you going into a physical incarnation?

ST: Yes,

KL: Into which tribe?

ST: Anambah. It is interesting how on one continent there are struggles and then on the next continent, there are similar struggles, survival struggles. It is a hard life but a rewarding life in that compared to the life that humans live now in this year, we are, there is more reward, there is more connection with the tribe. It may be a harder life, but there's more respect for one another, for the land for the animals. There's more gratitude for the food.

KL: Are you male or female?

ST: I'm female.

KL: What is your name?

ST: Etaka.

KL: And how old are you Etaka?

ST: Again, I'm in my prime. I have a similar role, as you put it, shaman, healer, spirit keeper, connector.

KL: So, let's condense time and move forward to the next significant time. What's happening?

ST: I feel there is a terrible drought. People are losing hope, they fear that if the rains do not come soon, we will not survive. But I know the wisdom behind this. This is part of their learning if you like. They must learn to be more resourceful. They must learn to work more with the land although there is mutual respect they must learn to work more with the land. They must understand that this is a cycle it will pass. I feel people are losing hope. People are very hungry; they are beginning to turn on each other if you like. This again is a test. I understand this test. I try to reassure them. I try to keep the peace. There are some who do not wish to be in peace. I see that there is a separation. There is a divide that is beginning to appear. There are some who are planning to move on. Others wish to stay in hope that the rains will come as they do not wish to leave their homeland. There are others too, who are impatient, who do not trust that the rains are coming. They are very, very desperate. I had the faith that the rains will come.

KL: Have you been shown the rains?

ST: I just know that they will come.

KL: Let's move forward and see what happens next.

ST: So those people moved on. The village has now been divided. I feel we are a very small population now. We are regrowing, creating crops. The rains did come.

KL: You were right to have faith.

ST: I feel many would have perished in their journey. Those who left perished, many perished, many died, it has created a divide, it has created tension between the two. I feel because of this there is bloodshed. The man, the one they follow is very angry. He wishes to seek justice for those who lost their lives. You see there are many lessons that are being learnt, many tests, many initiations. I see that I feel that.

KL: Who do they want to seek justice from?

ST: Those who stayed those who he feels but did not give them the knowledge. He blames the elders. So, we have been divided.

KL: So, what happens now that you are divided?

ST: There is much tension.

KL: It's almost like two different tribes.

ST: Yes. This is a shame because we once lived in peace.

KL: It's very sad, so, what happens next?

ST: Many years of bloodshed. Things feel they will never be the same. We are constantly in fear of being attacked. I fear they will never stop until they seek justice.

KL: Do you have family Etaka?

ST: No. Not children.

KL: Do you have a wife? Yes.

KL: What's her name?

ST: Mia.

KL: So just take a moment to look into Mia's eyes and see if there's any recognition for anybody, that Sonya maybe knows in this lifetime.

ST: Yes, it's my son.

KL: Let's move forward and see what happens next.

ST: There is still unrest, we are thriving, food is abundant, growing in numbers doing some retry Life is good apart from the tension This is just the way things will be. We go out hunting for food and we come across the other tribe, there is always tension. Who will get the kill first? Whereas before we lived in peace, we would share the kill and eat together in harmony. You see, everybody needs to learn to relearn harmony, peace, unity. This is their lesson. We need to come together. I feel eventually this will happen. There will be much suffering.

KL: So, let's condense time and move forward and see what's happening. Do you find peace with the tribe? Does that peace come in your lifetime? What happens?

ST: The beginnings of it in my very old age when the white man comes into the village.

KL: Do you know what year it is now?

ST: 17 something. I'm not sure.

KL: So, the white man comes into the village, and then what happens?

ST: This creates tension between the white man, and I feel we are becoming united with the other tribe. The white man's presence makes us all feel uneasy.

KL: What is it that makes you feel uneasy about the white man's presence?

ST: They are very different from us.

KL: In what way?

ST: The way that they conduct themselves is very different. In a way, it is a blessing in that it has brought the tribes closer together, but they are creating a sense of unease within the groups. I feel they have a motive. They wish to control, divide, separate.

KL: So, let's move forward and see if you're right. What happens next?

ST: Well, I was right. The White Man is causing trouble. They want us to move on. We do not wish to move on. This is our land, our sacred land where our ancient brothers and sisters have lived upon this land. This is something we all have in common.

KL: Can you describe the land? Is it rocky or is it a valley? What's the landscape like?

ST: It's very green pastures, it's fertile.

KL: Is it flat?

ST: No, it's slightly hilly hills.

KL: What would we call this part of America now? Sonya may know.

ST: I'm not sure but I'm just. Arizona? I'm not sure.

KL: Etaka what happens next?

ST: There are many years of unrest. Many years of divide, many years of bloodshed. Many years of discussion, peace talks. We feel they will never give up. They will never stop.

KL: So, let's move forward just condensing time and see what happens. We'll move forward to the end of your life unless there's anything significant before then.

ST: Nothing much has changed. There's still unrest. They have restricted us. We're only allowed in certain parts of the land. They don't allow us to go further. Which is creating starvation. We're unable to hunt further afield. There are borders, they've created borders. We are unable to cross these borders.

KL: What would happen if you did cross them? Have people tried?

ST: They would take us and generally, you would never return.

KL: So, let's move forward and see what happens.

ST: It is my time to pass.

KL: How do you pass?

ST: Through old age. My body is very old. Not much has changed. Only that we've learned to adapt to our restricted life.

KL: So, let's move forward so that you can look back at that life out of the body. What were you learning from that lifetime?

ST: It was a collective learning to live together. Collectively learning to hold the peace, to be the peace.

KL: You're learning to hold the peace.

ST: My own personal journey was to learn more about humanity. They very much wish to control one another;

they struggle to live as a unit to pace there is the need for possession.

KL: I wonder what the Lords of light have to say to humanity currently.

ST: No civilization goes through the journey simply. There will always be struggle, there will always be divide. For this is balance. It's how you approach one another, how you interact with one another, the journey. With evolution comes devolution. One step forward, two steps back. It is learning to create that balance of taking one step forward, and then another step forward, then another step instead of continuously backstepping. With your technology, you step forward but as a collective race, you step back. And it is learning to balance these two polarities.

KL: I wonder what it would take, it seems to be that the leaders of our countries call the shots.

ST: They are those who create instability.

KL: How are we to break that instability? I'm sure that there are a lot of humanity that are quite happy to live together peacefully, called service.

ST: This is where balance comes into force.

KL: So, what can humanity do to create balance and conscious leadership?

ST: Humanity will collectively unite to balance out these negativities. There will always be negativity in balance. But it is learning to rise above, to negate, to be strong, to stand in their own power.

KL: Do you think that this is what the protesters are doing?

ST: They are creating a wave of justice. They are creating the wave for others to follow. They can see this imbalance, this injustice and within them is this force that wishes to expose those negative forces. You could say that that is the tidal wave.

KL: Do you have any other guidance for humanity currently?

ST: Think with the heart, not with the mind. If the collective thought with the heart and not with the mind, life would be very, very different. It is such a simple way of living. Many do not think with the heart, feel the heart. They are coming from the place of the mind. Just having greater thought for all of humanity, the planet, taking responsibility for everything. Individually taking responsibility, you could say that the seeds have been planted throughout the globe. The seedlings are beginning to appear. This is what you would describe as the awakening. When people perceive life, from the space in the heart, there will be peace, there will be love.

KL: Well, I wonder how long that will take?

ST: It is a very long journey.

Reflections

I then called in the higher self to see if there were any further messages for the client. I downloaded the lessons, blessings, and gifts for the client before bringing her out of trance.

This was once again a wonderful session, providing great insight and wisdom for the client, and again interesting information for humanity.

Future Life Progression

As I have said, there is no time, no past, present, and future, effectively it's all happening now. Future life progression can include the immediate future or longer-term future on earth and/or parallel/multi-dimensional lives in other realms and dimensions on other planets. Often, I will use it with clients to help them access insight, guidance, and resources from their future self and thus enable them to step into their highest timeline by retrieving gifts and abilities. There are many ways that we can utilise future life progression. Often, I will use it with clients to help them access insight, guidance, and resources from their future self and thus enable them to step into their highest timeline by retrieving and embodying future gifts and abilities. This work is highly transformational as clients can create a more positive self-identity, transform unwanted thoughts, feelings, behaviours, gain insight and information on new solutions, inventions, and look at various choices and what their potentials are.

Many of the women I work with are struggling with low self-worth, low self-image, self-esteem, doubt, imposter syndrome, lack of confidence, they struggle to up-level their business, yet when they connect with their future self, they feel more aligned with their vision because they're more powerful, confident, have high self-esteem and high self-worth, they've overcome their challenges, they've taken inspired action and they're now living their dreams and enjoying the happiness, success, and fulfilment that comes from aligning with your heart and soul's vision. As there is no time, and we create our reality, we can change our future, and thus all future information is a probability. When we see something in our future, if we make a different decision, or choose another path, we literally change our future. When we connect with the 'future life' and embrace and embody the future self, we collapse timelines and literally jump and quantum leap into our highest timeline.

In hypnosis, clients may go into a future galactic life and receive information for the planet and humanity. Many times, in meditation with galactic star-beings, I have been given information on personal and collective issues regarding the future, that have come true. Some of my prophetic insight comes true in a week or two, others may be further ahead. In 2018 I was in meditation with the Star Lions from Sirius and was told, 'Rome, Washington DC, London, the redistribution of wealth'. I was also shown the Olympic Games circles. I was expecting the stock exchange to go down but didn't know when. It wasn't until the information regarding the Covid 19 Virus came out as having started in Wuhan, China, where the 2019 Military World Games took place, that I realised what they were talking about and why I was shown the Olympic circles and then of course the stock market went down 40%.

You can also go into a Theta Brain Wave, expand out beyond the edge of the universe, and ask your Higher Self or Source, what happened last time I took this action? This is a powerful tool, that I use a lot and it brings great awareness of future events and possibilities. I only wish that I'd remembered to use this tool when flying back from

Montana a few years back. I was travelling with a friend, and we forgot to go up and see the future before travelling home and we ended up missing our flight. Despite the plane still being on the ground, we were not allowed to board and had to spend a thousand pounds on another flight. We live and learn!

If you see a future event that you don't like, you can ask what would it take to change this? How can I create the most beneficial outcome for myself, for others and the planet? What else is possible? Your future self might show you the choice points that led to this future and how and where you might choose differently.

Mary & Ann Boleyn Execution & A Possible Future Life

In this session, my client wanted to work on visibility issues. She is a holistic therapist and teacher and was ready to up-level her business but found herself unable to be visible on social media. She lacked confidence in being on video and had a fear of being criticised and just couldn't bring herself to show up fully online. I work with a lot of spiritual healers, therapists, and entrepreneurs and this is a very common theme. Often this is linked with fear of persecution, fear of being judged, imposter syndrome, feeling like a fraud. These issues may be rooted in the current life, there may be ancestral issues and of course, they can be rooted in past lives. Often, it's a combination of all three. In past lives, often this can link with past lives where the client was persecuted, accused or on trial or may simply come from a life where they were criticised either in this life or in a past life, or on the ancestral level. In this session, the client first was taken into an incident in her childhood, before going into a past life. Where she was taken to Ann Boleyn's Execution, and then that very quickly shifted to another life that felt like she was back in the past and at the same time appeared to her to be in the future. Each session is unique and truly a wonderful mystery tour.

ST: So, I've gone back to my childhood when I was at secondary school, and the anxiety and the fear around, standing up in class and speaking or reading or something, it's making me feel quite anxious.

KL: Okay. And so, let's see what happened. You're feeling anxious, how old are you?

ST: 13 or 14.

KL: Who's there? Is there a teacher there?

ST: I know that a teacher would be there, but I'm not seeing the teacher. It's just me experiencing that memory of how it felt.

KL: Okay, so just allow yourself to feel that feeling for a moment. Where in your body do you feel that?

ST: It's in my stomach.

KL: So, just allow that feeling in your stomach to take you deeper and deeper into that experience, to the place this anxiety and fear of being seen, fear of speaking up first began.

ST: So now, I've just flashed into another life where I was Mary Boleyn and I'm experiencing similar feelings, but this is more about me being seen. I want to say, by the vultures. I'm feeling very anxious about being around people in court. I don't want to be there. I don't want to be seen. It's like a fear of being seen because I'm a female. I don't want that sort of attention.

KL: What will happen if you're seen?

ST: Well, I'll probably have no choice but to fulfil the desires of those in power.

KL: What will you have to do if you must fulfil the desires of those in power?

ST: I don't really want to. I'm far too young. I don't want to be in that situation.

KL: How old are you?

ST: A number just came in my head, and it was 13.

KL: And when you say that you'd have to fulfil their desires. What does that mean?

ST: So, if a pretty, young girl comes into court, she's new, she's attractive. She's seen; you know there's a desire there from others. They may want to fulfil their urges,

KL: Their sexual urges, you mean?

ST: Yes.

KL: Okay. So, you fear men desiring you?

ST: Yes. But not just that, I just don't want to be here. I just don't want to be seen. I don't want to be in this place. But I don't really have much choice.

KL: Why do you not have many choices?

ST: Because of the family lines. It's just what we must do. We must follow the family lines.

KL: So, Mary, let's move forward to a significant time and see what happens.

ST: I know this timeline. This is Ann's execution. I was standing at the back, watching. I have a black coat with a hood on and black gloves. I'm standing at the back, watching. I wasn't supposed to be there. I feel guilty that I could have done more to prevent what happened.

KL: How old are you?

ST: I'm a young woman. I don't know. Barely in my 20s, not sure, something like that.

KL: And who is it that's got the black cloak on?

ST: That's me.

KL: Okay. So, you're wearing a black cloak and black gloves. And what's Ann wearing?

ST: She's wearing a velvet dress. It's plain. It's quite low, low, so they can get to the neck. They make them like that. Short sleeves. It's very basic. I believe it's a dark colour.

KL: And what is your relationship with Ann?

ST: She is my sister.

KL: And how are you feeling?

ST: Helpless.

KL: And who else is there that you know?

ST: Nobody. I'm on my own. Well, there are lots of people here, but I'm not supposed to be there. I have this big hood on, which is why I am hiding and covering my face.

KL: What do you think would happen if people saw you?

ST: Well, it was forbidden because of the shame upon the family.

KL: Who forbade it?

ST: My father, my mother, the court. It's very sad.

KL: So why is she being executed?

ST: She played a very, very dangerous game. And you know what? I saw it coming. I knew that this would backfire.

KL: What did she do?

ST: She was playing games within courts. She was very flirtatious around other men. She just wanted danger the whole time. She had to fill this dangerous thrill.

KL: So, let's move forward and see what happens.

ST: So, I am no longer part of the court, and I was at the execution, which is why it was easy for me to get there. I am no longer part of it. I've moved away. I have my own home, which I'm happy with. I'm very happy in my home.

KL: Where do you live? What's your home like?

ST: It's a beautiful manor house in the countryside.

KL: Wonderful. So, has Ann been executed now?

ST: Yes.

KL: Let's move forward, and let's see if there's anything significant in this lifetime, allowing any scenes to close in three, two, one, finding yourself in another scene, another time.

ST: I'm playing in a field with my son. He's very happy. He's giggling and laughing. He must be about seven or eight. It's just him and I.

KL: What's your son's name?

ST: Edward?

KL: Where is your husband?

ST: He's not with us. He's around, but not with us.

KL: So, you're playing in the field?

ST: Yeah, it's just a beautiful moment. The sun is bright. It's such a lovely warm day, and there's a slight breeze, and the grass is blowing in the wind. It's just really a lovely moment.

KL: And is there anything else significant here for you or should we move forward? (Move forward) Ok so let's move forward, finding yourself leaving that scene moving forward to another time, another space—a place that's significant.

As this scene closes, the client now moves into another life.

ST: I'm back to when we first went into the meditation. I'm standing on a very tall hill or a very rural mountain. I'm dressed in what look like Ugg boots. They're not; they're made of sheepskin and fur.

KL: Are you male or female?

ST: I'm female.

KL: What's your name?

ST: I'm not sure.

KL: Okay. Just look down at your feet. And then you can move up your body and see what else you're wearing.

ST: So, the boots look very Native American. I have a bow and arrow.

KL: Very good. So, look around you at the landscape and see where you are.

ST: I'm so high up, and you can see for miles and miles and miles, and there's this thick black fog over the landscape.

KL: Are you on a mountain?

ST: Yeah, I must be by how high I am. But there are lots and lots of rolling hills. It's interesting because it doesn't look like America; it looks like England.

KL: Okay, so just allowing your conscious mind, to simply relax and let go, allowing yourself to go deeper and deeper into this experience. So, you're on this mountain; you're looking out at these beautiful rolling hills. How are you feeling?

ST: Well, a couple of words are coming to my head. Settlement. I'm seeing what kind of looks like yurts. It's like I'm looking down at the settlement. They live in yurts.

KL: Are you living in a yurt?

ST: I'm not sure.

KL: So, let's see what happens.

ST: So, I'm starting to run down the hillside and the fog has cleared, and there are beautiful flowers like little white daisies.

KL: Beautiful. What else can you see? Are there people?

ST: I don't see anyone else here now. I'm now next to a river. A little river that's running through woodland.

KL: What kind of trees are there?

ST: They're very mossy; their trunks have green moss on them. Again, it looks like English woodland. This river looks very manmade. It's like somebody has purposely put all these rocks there to direct this water, and the bed of the river is lots and lots of little pebbles. It's not a natural one when I say it's not really a river. It's more like a little brook. But I feel this has been manmade.

KL: If you were to know what year it was? Perhaps you can see the numbers written on the floor. Just the first number that comes into your mind.

ST: Well, I think I'm trying to analyse it. The first number that came into my head was 18.

KL: Ok, let's move forward and see what happens.

ST: I'm now foraging and hunting. I'm hunting a deer. I'm stalking this deer in the woods. Our yurts are made of animal hide. What is bizarre is that I've just gone over a stile. A wooden stile that you would get now. It looks like it's rotten and old.

KL: Okay, let's see what happens.

ST: So, I'm just entering a field, and this field is very much the type of field that you would see in somewhere like Cornwall, where they use rocks to build the boundaries.

KL: Like dry stone walls. Very good, so let's see what you're doing here. Are you still stalking the deer?

ST: No, the deer have gotten away. I feel guided to go over to one of the brick walls and pull out a brick and inside is a gold chain with a round locket.

KL: Is there anything in the locket?

ST: I believe there's a picture of a family member in this locket, and I can't help but think that this is the future. I don't believe this is the past. I think I'm seeing the future.

KL: Okay, so let's open the locket and see inside.

ST: I think it's my mum. (My brain is trying to analyse this all.)

KL: So just allow your unconscious mind to step aside and allow each and every breath you take to take you deeper and deeper, more and more relaxed, that's right, deeper now into that wonderful deep relaxation.

ST: I feel that anything that is precious like that you need to hide.

KL: For what reason?

ST: Because I feel that there's not a lot of this around, that people don't have gold chains. This is something that is quite rare.

KL: Do you know what year it is?

ST: I'm having problems identifying that. What I'm getting is 18, but I don't know what the first two numbers are.

KL: If you were to imagine those two numbers, what numbers come into your mind now? You can make it up if you like.

ST: I think it's a three.

KL: So, is it 318?

ST: I think it's 301, which would be crazy.

KL: Let's move forward and see what happens next.

ST: So, I've gone back with the rest of the people. There aren't many people living within this community.

KL: Do you have family here?

ST: I don't feel like I do.

KL: Is there something significant for you to see at this time?

ST: I feel that when I compare this lifetime with my current life, it may appear on the surface that we've gone backwards. It is so different. It's like I've gone back hundreds and hundreds of years. It's the future time. We have everything we need, food shelter, warmth. But I don't see any of the technologies that we have now. When I was standing on that mountainside, all I could see was just rolling hills and fields. I couldn't see any other settlements, any other people. It's like there's no one else around in this area.

KL: How many people are in this settlement with you?

ST: I want to say six.

KL: So, it's a very small settlement.

ST: Yes.

KL: And are any of those people family to you?

ST: No.

KL: Let's move forward and see what happens.

ST: I sense that I'm at some stone structures like Stonehenge, something similar.

KL: When you say a stone structure, what kind of format does it have? Is it a circle?

ST: Yeah, it looks very much like Stonehenge. I feel that there has been a pilgrimage to this place.

KL: Are there others with you?

ST: Yes, but a very, very small group.

KL: And what is the purpose of this pilgrimage?

ST: Because it's a sacred site.

KL: What time of year is it?

ST: Well, I don't feel cold. It's weird, but there's no one else there. I don't believe we've met anyone else on our travels either.

KL: What do you do at the sacred site?

ST: We've just come here just to be in this place. Just to be in the energy of the stones.

KL: How do you feel in this place? How do you feel when you touch the stones? How do you feel being in this sacred site?

ST: I don't really feel anything.

KL: Are you happy to be here?

ST: Yes.

KL: Ok, let's move forward and see what happens.

ST: This is weird. I'm now under the ice; it's like a big ice tunnel. It's beautiful. It's like got this lovely blue haze, and the shapes are amazing. I'm still wearing those same boots and the same clothes. With what I'm wearing, it seems more fitting with the temperature.

KL: Are you dressed for the cold?

ST: Yeah, but I've always been dressed in an old sheepskin coat that goes down to my boots and a big hood. I'm wearing that now.

KL: So, you're under the ice tunnel?

ST: Yeah, we're just looking for people. At the bottom of the base of this tunnel, there's a little river and we're walking in the river. All around us is this ice tunnel.

KL: How did you get into the ice tunnel?

ST: I've got no idea, I don't know.

KL: Looking through the tunnel, how deep is this water at the base of the tunnel?

ST: Very shallow. It's a constant flow of water.

KL: So, I wonder, do you find any other people?

ST: Well, we haven't done so far; maybe that's what we're looking for.

KL: Do you have any memory of your family?

ST: I'm not sure. If I do, it feels very distant. I can't help but think that I never ever met my mom, which is why that locket is so important to me.

KL: So, do you know what happened to your mum?

ST: I want to say that she perished.

KL: What about your father?

ST: I don't know anything about him.

KL: So, let's condense time and let's move forward to the end of this time and see what happens.

ST: I just see water; it's very choppy water.

KL: Is it the river or the sea? What type of water is it?

ST: It's the sea. There appear to be a lot of whales in the sea. I'm in a little boat on my own. I'm hanging on for dear life because it's so choppy, and I don't have any oars or anything.

KL: What's the boat made of?

ST: The boat's made of wood.

KL: Let's move forward and see what happens. What happens next?

ST: I'm not sure what's happening now.

KL: Are you in a body?

ST: I don't know.

KL: Let's call in your highest self, that part of you that's always aware. You showed us the lifetime of Mary Boleyn. And then you showed us the lifetime of the settlement.

ST: It was to show you the insignificance of those lifetimes in terms of the struggle, the worry. The soul is infinite, and those lifetimes were a very short proportion of the whole.

KL: And I wonder if there's a significance about Sonya's fears or anxieties about being visible. In those lifetimes, she felt anxious about men's desires, and she witnessed an execution, and she said that she said she thought she had to hide things that were precious. What's stopping her from being visible now in this lifetime?

ST: Fear of judgement.

KL: How can you best help Sonya to overcome this? What's the worst thing about being judged?

ST: That others would say unkind words.

KL: Why is it the worst thing if someone did say unkind words?

ST: It would knock her off balance.

KL: Is there something that you can do to help her with it?

ST: Future timelines are opening. It is a matter of facing fear. When one is visible, one must expect others to not understand because not everybody will be understanding of the teachings; some of them are not ready yet, some do not understand. So, when they analyse and make judgments, it is not because of malice; it is because people do not understand they have not yet evolved.

KL: Yeah. So, can we teach Sonya what it feels like to live without the fear of others' criticism or judgement? What's the feeling that she needs so that she can be able to be seen without fearing that criticism and judgement from others?

ST: To not take rejection so personally. It's not a reflection of her actions or abilities. To think of the whole, not just, oh, I am not worthy of this.

KL: Well, thank you very much for showing Sonya those lifetimes and perhaps if there are any feelings that you might like to download to Sonya or anything that you wish her to have that she doesn't have, or any resources that you can download now or later. Knowing that you're always in communication with your highest self and that these lessons can be received in the highest and the best way possible for you.

ST: I would like to add something. When we analyse the lives that have been shown, the last life, there was no judgement, there was no being in view, being seen. And it was to demonstrate that these experiences are familiar. If we tap into those past experiences, they can assist us in this current lifetime.

KL: Yes, that's true. There is always something that we can learn and benefit from. Let's bring your body and cellular memory up to date with all of that, so that you know the difference between then and now.

Reflections

During the integration process, the client connected with her higher self, who referred to her fear of judgment and rejection that were connected with her current visibility issues, giving wonderful advice. She learnt that it's safe for her to share her most treasured gifts with the world.

Our connection with our higher self is a wonderful resource to gain insight, guidance, and advice both personally and also within our business. Connecting with the Higher Self is one of the first things that I do with my clients to empower them to go within and receive inner guidance. With practice, it's possible to learn how to channel your Higher Self and again this is something that I teach my clients to do. Channelling is a wonderful skill that can be used not only for personal guidance, insight, wisdom, and healing but also for business guidance, developing your business ideas, writing business marketing materials and so much more. Most of us are unconsciously channelling our soul's desires when we are happy and aligned with our heart and doing what we love, expressing our heart and soul. Many refer to this way of living as following their soul's purpose.

China Dam-Future Interplanetary Life

In this session, my client was interested in connecting with a future life. There are many ways that we can utilise future life progression. Often, I will use it with clients to help them access insight, guidance, and resources from their future self and thus enable them to step into their highest timeline by retrieving gifts and abilities. As always, the client's higher self is guiding the session and the session took an interesting direction.

(Client swallows)

KL: Where are you now?

ST: I can see a big dam. This dam is huge, it's a massive, huge dam, and it feels like there are too many people on the earth. Far too many people.

KL: Okay, do you know where this dam is?

ST: China?

KL: So, why does it feel like there are too many people on the earth?

ST: There's so much confusion.

KL: Are you in a body?

ST: Yes.

KL: So just take a look down at your feet and notice what you're wearing on your feet.

ST: Shimmering shoes.

KL: What else are you wearing?

ST: I'm wearing something like a shield over my face.

KL: What type of shield is it?

ST: Like a glass face shield that covers my face. I'm wearing a shimmering bodysuit. I don't believe I'm from this earth. I think I've come back to visit, to observe.

KL: Oh, where are you from then?

ST: Many places, Venus. We've lived in many places.

KL: When you say we, who are you referring to?

ST: We, the observers, have come to observe what is happening on the earth. Humanity is coping with the new reality that is presenting itself to them.

KL: Do you have a name?

ST: Shiana. I feel that that is the easiest translation.

KL: Are you female, Shiana?

ST: Yes.

KL: And the dam in China, is that you in the future life?

ST: That is me coming back to observe.

KL: So, you're coming back to visit earth in your shimmery shoes and your shimmery suit, and is that Shiana?

ST: Yes. I do not live on earth. I have come back to assist.

KL: You're saying that there are too many people on earth? What is it about the dam that is significant?

ST: It is significant because this was part of humanity's awakening, part of their understanding of what their future held.

KL: I wonder if you can help in terms of what year it is on earth?

ST: It's 2060. What has happened is a natural progression for the earth, but it has been accelerated, and humanity has been warned many times, but they did not listen. They chose not to listen.

KL: How do you feel about that?

ST: Very sad because it could have been avoided if they had listened.

KL: Right. So, from where we are now, you're talking about 40 years into the future, from our perspective on the earth. How long have you been observing?

ST: Always. We have always been observing. We are many.

KL: Does Shiana have an earth body in 2060?

ST: I don't know.

KL: Okay. So, tell us about the dam. What's the significance of the dam? What happens next?

ST: The dam is preventing the water from rising, from flooding, villages, towns, cities, but it will only hold for a short period of time, and eventually, the dam will give way. I feel so sad.

KL: You say this is because people haven't listened.

ST: Yes.

KL: Is there anything that people can do? If you were to give people advice now, what advice would you give to humanity to be able to change? Or is that not a possibility?

ST: Humanity has the answers. They know the answers. They do not wish to listen. There is much that can be done to prevent this catastrophic disaster.

KL: Is there more that you wish to say about that, or do you want to move forward?

ST: I would like to add that there are pockets of beings in humanity who did listen and who prophesied that this would happen. We would like to add that this is a possible timeline. There are other timelines. You could say at present, humanity is on the cusp of… they are at the edge of the cliff. It is their choice as to whether they listen or they don't listen. This is a possible timeline that could occur.

KL: Yes. As you say, there are many timelines. So, if the dam breaks, can you tell us what is ahead on that timeline?

ST: Many lives will be lost.

KL: From a global perspective, what will be the implications of that dam breaking? Is it something that's local to China or...?

ST: This is throughout the whole of the earth.

KL: So, there are other places where there are floods?

ST: Yes.

KL: Is there more that you wish to say at this time?

ST: No.

KL: You said we, can I just ask about your family, your planet? Do you work as a group consciousness or...?

ST: We are many diverse beings, we come from many planets. We come together to assist humanity.

KL: I see. Are you living on a planet at the moment, or do you have a ship? How does that work?

ST: I feel we are hovering above earth. I see light, bright light.

KL: So, you said that you were in the eighth dimension, is that right? Can you describe your body? You have spoken of your sparkly suit, sparkly, shimming shoes. They sound very beautiful.

ST: I can show myself in whatever way I wish to be seen.

KL: Are you able to describe how that works? The process of being able to show yourself in any way you wish.

ST: Thought materialization.

KL: So, you don't have a physical body, but you use your thoughts, and you materialize, and you form a body.

ST: Yes.

KL: Yes. How does that process of being able to create a body serve you? Why do you do that?

ST: I do this to please the recipient.

KL: So, they can recognize you and connect with you?

ST: Yes.

KL: How do you communicate with them?

ST: Telepathically?

KL: Is that how you communicate with your own people?

ST: Yes.

KL: Thank you for explaining that process. Have you been to Earth before?

ST: Yes.

KL: So, can you talk more about that? There are many questions that people have about the creation of humanity and those that have visited, and there are many stories. Could you share more about that?

ST: Yes, there is. Much misinformation. The earth was a rich planet, full of life. Many planets go through the same process. I'm trying to find the words that will make it sound less mechanical. You may think it is a little mechanical. We wish to expand life, to enhance life; it's like having a child. You feel pride; you feel love for that child. You see them grow into wonderful adults. They are part of your creation. It is very similar. All creation takes place with love. We wish to expand life, for life is truly diverse. Humanity sees a small portion of the diversity of life within the solar system. So, the earth was part of this creation process. Where life was impregnated upon the earth, and this evolved with the assistance of others over many, thousands of years. I believe you understand that man did not suddenly evolve to his current specification. This was a creation. We want the best. We want humans to fly, to evolve, to become the best possible version of themselves. The earth was very different when we first came here. Through many, many visitations, life evolved, and it was very beautiful, it was lush, it was green, rivers, oceans, cascading crystal-clear water, animals, birds, it was a thriving ecosystem, it was beautiful.

KL: It sounds idyllic.

ST: It was. So, it was ripe for the next phase of the creation—to create a life form. I have to be very careful of the words that I use.

KL: Oh, why's that?

ST: I feel that I have to be very careful with the information that I am disclosing to you.

KL: Well, I trust that you can find the right words and the right information.

ST: The human is birthed in love. Everything we do is created from love. Is always done because of love.

KL: I understand that, though not everybody would see it or understand it in that way.

ST: You see, we see your future timelines and wish the best for you all. Much of humanity has struggled to understand the evolution of life.

KL: There are many theories.

ST: Because they do not understand. It is beyond their current capable understanding. So, they created a version that was acceptable to your collective. An understandable version that could be understood by many.

KL: Well, there are many stories. I'm wondering if you're referring to the Bible story.

ST: Yes.

KL: Can I ask you about any genetic manipulation?

ST: This is part of the process.

KL: Is this something that you feel comfortable speaking about? Or is this what you're having to be careful of speaking about?

ST: I can disclose some of the information.

KL: That would be helpful.

ST: So, if we take a tadpole, that tadpole grows, evolves, grows little legs, little arms, it loses its tail, it grows into a frog. So, with every process of evolution that that tadpole that frog goes through, we are able to assist in a positive way, so that frog becomes the best possible version it could be. Through genetic manipulation, through combining other species into its genetic makeup. So, it becomes the best possible version of itself in every possible way.

KL: So much of humanity at this time, or a portion of humanity, have questions around the genetic manipulation, around the reptilian energy. I wonder if you might like to talk more about Reptilian energy.

ST: I feel there is much negativity towards the reptilian energy, and it is unnecessary. You must understand that every species within the cosmos has gone through its evolution. Much like humans, they have made mistakes, they have evolved, they have ascended, but ultimately, there was always love there. I do not feel that there has been any malice or intentional damage to humanity by this race. You must understand that when you look from the bigger picture, you see it from so many perspectives, for when you just see from the one perspective, it is very linear. When you look from the collective, from the higher aspect, you see the situation very, very differently. That is some of what humanity is currently learning, evolving, understanding. When they see things so linear, they do not see things from the wider perspective, the wider understanding. I see a beautiful blue planet. I feel that I have moved to this beautiful blue planet.

KL: This beautiful blue planet that you see, can you tell us where it is? Does it have a name?

ST: Sirius. It is very dear to my heart.

KL: Have you lived there at some point?

ST: Yes.

KL: What did you most love about Sirius?

ST: It was such a beautiful planet? Many fond moments were spent with my beautiful brothers and sisters. Many diverse beings and it is very blue, very different from earth. You see, it is not necessary to have such physical beauty, for we can create our own beauty. It's like a crystal, like a diamond.

KL: Is there a reason that it's a diamond?

ST: Because it has so many facets, clear. It's just a beautiful, beautiful planet.

KL: What kinds of beings? We talked about your brothers and sisters, but what kind of other beings?

ST: An example is my beautiful friend; he is a bird being, and he's blue.

KL: Does he have a name?

ST: That is difficult. He is a traveller; he travels.

KL: Is he what would we call a Blue Avian?

ST: If that is what you would like to refer to him as. He's blue; he's bird-like.

KL: There are so many stories and so many questions that would take us months and years. So, is there anything significant that you could share with us about the blue avian race and their connection with humanity? Do they have a different role for you?

ST: Collectively, we all have the same role—to assist, to be ready. We await in the wings. We work with many of you, some, unknowingly, to raise the vibration to assist, guide and nurture. We are very fond of humanity.

KL: I have many questions, and I'm trying to allow you to speak without interrupting you.

ST: I'm travelling.

KL: Where are we travelling to next?

ST: Everything is yellow. We are ascending to the Lords of Light.

KL: Does your planet have a name?

ST: Delta.

KL: Delta? Is there some other name that we would know? Many of our constellations have stars called Delta.

ST: It is to the higher level of consciousness. The beings have evolved.

KL: When you say beings, what beings? Are you referring to the Sirians, or is this another planet?

ST: These are beyond that. I refer to them as the Lords of Light.

KL: Thank you for clarifying.

ST: It's difficult to explain. They are the purest highest level of consciousness.

KL: What dimension would they be?

ST: I don't know whether I can explain it to you. For you understand dimensions 1, 2, 3, 4, 5 and so on, and they are beyond dimensions. They are everything. They are space; they are time. They are all of creation.

KL: Are they what we refer to as the Gods?

ST: I do not wish to mislead you. They are a similar force.

KL: Do we know them as the Elohim?

ST: They are similar. Everything is light. Their energy, their consciousness, is in everything from the smallest particle to the ocean, to the stars to the planets; they are part of everything.

KL: I wonder if you can talk about that process of Ascension. Before they ascended, did they have a dimension?

ST: They were everything.

KL: So, they were everything before they ascended to the laws of light?

ST: They were everything. They were the dimensions; there is no separation.

KL: Sometimes, we talk about planes rather than dimensions.

ST: Levels of evolution. Yeah.

KL: So, did they move to another plane when they ascended?

ST: They are everything.

KL: Are we all everything?

ST: We are part of everything, okay. But we are not everything.

KL: And when we ascend, we become more of everything and more of who we become?

ST: We merge with the greater creation, which is beyond your current understanding.

KL: Tell us more about the Lords of Light.

ST: They emanate such peace and love. They are pure. They are the force of all creation. They emanate in everything. They are the creators. They are not physical beings. They are a force. They are in everything. They are in the heart of every being. This is what creates the pull to go home. When two magnets meet, there is a pull. You naturally want to gravitate towards that place—complete peace, stillness, joy, euphoria. You just lose yourself in their expanse.

KL: Can you talk a little bit about when you just lose yourself in their expanse? I'm wondering if you can talk about the differences or similarities between group consciousness and individuality. So many people think that when they ascend, they will have group consciousness, one mind, and they'll lose their individuality. So have the Lords of Light lost their individuality, or do they have a group consciousness?

ST: They did not lose anything. All creation wishes to be a part of that expanse as they evolve to greater awareness. Greater consciousness, they become closer to this expanse. It's like a beacon, a beacon of light to which you naturally are attracted to. This is part of the journey of life. All life is on a journey. It's a journey of awareness, connection, life. It all leads to the same place—an unseen force but knowing that it exists. Such beauty.

KL: So beautiful.

ST: We all have it within us; it's part of the soul's journey to find that expanse. To be part of that expanse. To merge with that expanse, and from that expanse, there is life.

ST: I'm back on earth now, standing next to the dam. That was lovely.

KL: Well, that was an interesting trip around the world in 80 days. Around the Solar System, really, around the galaxy.

ST: Yeah, I have many friends that I connect with.

Reflection

This was a wonderful session where the client went to a future or parallel life and received interesting information regarding a possible future event on Earth. Remember, when we are looking at future timelines, they are probabilities. Our future is not laid in stone, but created with every choice and step we take.

Spirit Attachment & Spirit Release

Before we move on to talk about spirit attachment and spirit release, let me share with you a little background.

You have no doubt heard of spirit attachments, or entities, these are various beings who are discarnate, no longer in a body. Usually, when we die, we would go to the light, but some spirits get stuck in between realms. This may be due to a sudden or traumatic passing, unresolved issues they want to address, they don't know that they've died, they're scared to go to the light, or they have attachment or addictions that cause them to want to hang around the earth plane so they can continue their addictive tendencies. Discarnate spirit attachments can cause all kinds of issues when they attach to our aura and can affect our thoughts, feelings, behaviours, our body, creating illness, discomfort, pain and change in personality. Spirit release therapy offers us a process for clearing our body and energy field of all and any spirit attachments.

What is Spirit Attachment?

Spirit attachment often happens when a soul fails to go to the light when they die. This can happen for a number of reasons, here are some of the most common ones.

- A sudden or shocking death.
- Unresolved business with someone on the earth.
- Attached to the earth or earthly desires.

- Wanting to watch over someone (often family, loved ones, ancestors).
- Mistaken identity (the spirit thinks it's 'their' body).

Signs & Symptoms of a Spirit Attachment

There are many signs and symptoms of spirit attachment, and they vary drastically depending on the spirit, where and how and why they are attached to the person. A client may have some or several of these signs and symptoms. Some of the signs may be recent and drastic whilst others may not be so easily spotted as they may have been attached for some time and the person didn't notice.

- Feeling like you have a spirit attachment or are haunted.
- Feeling or experiencing the house where you live is haunted.
- Mental disorders like Schizophrenia and Schizo-affective disorder.
- Lethargy and feeling exhausted.
- Chronic, mystery, ongoing illness.
- Sudden onset of irritability, crankiness, or snappiness.
- Anger or rage issues not previously present.
- Anxiety, Fear, Panic Attacks, Depression.

- Sudden onset of Low Self Worth, Shame and Guilt, Drug or Alcohol Dependence.
- Frequent nausea or stomach illness.
- Extreme and often dangerous mood fluctuations.
- Any sudden behavioural or personality change.
- A feeling of heaviness or pressure.
- Waking up to presences around you at night.
- Feeling like you're 'dragging' or being weighed down on a frequent basis.
- Developing new vices.
- A negative outlook on life that was not previously present.
- Feeling like you have low energy.
- Pain in specific areas of the body that has seemingly no other cause.
- Bizarre, haunting, and horrifying dreams.

If you're spiritually inclined, being able to see or feel the same spirit, again and again, is another sign. One who does not look or behave lovingly or compassionately, portrays deep, painful emotion when appearing to you, stands far away or comes in dreams only, and/or you have memories from childhood of this person.

People who are vulnerable to spirit attachment

- People who have strong emotions can attract spirits with similar strong emotions.
- People with addictions may attract spirits with addictions who want to continue to enjoy their old addiction. They feed off the feelings and psychic energy of the person they're attached to.
- Soldiers or people who have killed people may end up with spirit attachments as well as PTSD.
- Health care professionals working in mental health, hospitals, hospices, care homes, paramedics, funeral directors.
- Healers, therapists, lightworkers, mediums, children who have very bright auras – earth-bound spirits are often may be drawn to their light and wish to communicate or be crossed over to the spirit world.

How Your Shadow Attracts Your Experiences

Most people realise that their conscious mind can attract certain situations and experiences to them, but many don't realise that their shadow or unconscious mind can also attract situations and experiences. Attachments are simply another situation and experience and a lesson around personal sovereignty and being and standing in your own power and light and resolving issues.

Often when people are going through attachment or entity issues they can feel as though they are a victim, and they are being persecuted. The truth however is that on some level they have created or attracted these experiences in order to learn and grow.

Most attachments are a result of a client giving an entity permission or cooperating with them in some way, either explicitly or complicity by allowing the energy to remain with them consciously or unconsciously. (Through unconscious behaviours that allow entities to attach or from an unconscious need or desire which the entity meets)

Remember these energies can act like magnets to entities:

Drugs (incl. recreational and prescription drugs) and alcohol.

The use of drugs and alcohol can lower or impact your energetic vibration and auric field, resulting in vulnerability to attract low vibrational spirits.

Low-level emotions: anger, rage, shame, frustration, victim, grief etc. that are suppressed, repressed, or indeed unconsciously expressed or projected can and do attract low vibrational spirits.

Essentially, anything in your shadow is denied or repressed, so fears of evil and the dark side, vows to battle evil can and will subconsciously attract these experiences. Vows can be from current life, past lives, ancestral lives, spirit/soul (life between lives) 3D realm is a realm of duality, as is the 4D and lower 5D. Many healers, lightworkers, shamans have 5D beliefs and vows that cause issues connected with taking on clients' energies or battling evil. It's useful to muscle test and clear these issues, particularly if you are working as a healer, therapist and working therapeutically with clients.

It's important to know that we are all essentially one. On the higher planes of consciousness, there is no duality, no dark/light for all is serving the one. As Shakespeare said: *All the world's a stage and we are merely the players.*

It's also possible for people to unconsciously project their own shadow negativity and evil onto others or to obligate others to represent this energy for them, in order for them to see it and heal it. Many times, you will find when triggered by someone that it is simply your unconscious shadow within you that is seeking to be acknowledged and healed.

How and Why Spirits Can Attach to People: Kimberley's Case Notes

The following are some of my case notes, regarding spirit attachment and spirit release. Names have been changed.

Emma

Emma was an empath, highly kinaesthetic. She was concerned that she felt so much sadness, and that the sadness had been with her since childhood, despite a lot of personal growth work and clearing she had been unable to release the sadness that came up. In trance, she regressed to a three-year-old child, who was in her room crying. She identified a three-year-old girl called Bella who had befriended her at this time. (She had no conscious memory of this, although she did say that she had vivid dreams and a vivid imagination at this age and imaginary or spirit children playmates.)

In the session, the spirit child said that she wanted her mummy, that she hadn't meant to upset Emma but that she was waiting for her mummy, Bella shared that Emma had been her mother in a past life, we didn't manage to get any more information, the feeling was that the mother had died. Emma's inner child had been a playmate for this lonely sad spirit, their joint sadness had created a bond and as she grew in her personal development, Emma's adult self had been a mother figure for Bella as well as for her inner child.

I asked Emma's higher self if there were any soul fragments to be cleared. Higher self said Yes, please clear the soul fragments. The soul fragments were cleared, and I invited Emma and her inner three-year-old to tell the girl that she would be taken to find her mother, to say her goodbyes and we called in Mother Mary and Jesus to take her to find her mother in the spirit world. Emma then spoke with her inner child, who said that she was quite happy now, as she didn't want to leave the little girl alone.

We did some inner mother work with Emma's inner child and downloaded that she was safe, loved, supported, never alone. Mother Mary was there for her, and Emma was there for her. Emma's inner child said that she would love to have more fun. Emma is so serious at times and the inner child wanted to play. Emma admitted that she too wanted to have more fun and play in her life, so they began thinking of fun and playful things to do together.

Fiona

When I asked what happened 15 years ago when the problem started the client said her grandmother had died. The extraordinary thing was that the client herself had been an inpatient in the exact same hospital in a different hospital ward at the time! The Grandmother had simply zipped into the client instead of going to the light!

Once I had completed the spirit release and extraction the client felt much less heavy and less critical and exhausted, and the client's life improved considerably.

Jack

Jack lay on the massage couch eyes closed and I saw his eyes roll up into the top of his head, the whites of his eyes were showing, and I thought he might start spitting any minute! His ex-wife had cursed him. I had the client talk to his ex-wife, releasing any grief, sadness, shame, guilt, anger from the relationship, we released the curse and used a forgiveness process with his ex-wife and his children to resolve the situation, and call back soul fragments, releasing any quantum entanglements with his ex-wife and adult children and downloading all the lessons, blessings, and gifts from their relationship. Jack learned that he could forgive himself, he no longer needed to punish himself or obligate others to punish him, he claimed back his worth and power and his depression lifted.

Sally

My client had been psychic since childhood, in fact, her mother was also a psychic and clairvoyant. As a child, she had seen a ghost with an ugly face, who used to scare her so much she hid under the covers. Unfortunately, that ghost had attached to her. Once we communicated with the ghost, he disappeared, never to be seen again and my client was no longer frightened of the dark.

Shaun

Shaun had a marijuana habit and had been smoking heavily for some time, although he had recently stopped smoking marijuana, he began smoking cigarettes again and was smoking heavily. When scanning his body, I clairvoyantly saw something in his back, and in a trance when working with him around this issue we connected with wayward spirits who were connected with marijuana and cigarette use. When I asked him where in his body, the spirits were, they replied they could speak for themselves. They told me they were around his vertebrae, and they projected fear, stress, and a need for support, causing the client to continue to smoke. They enjoyed smoking, both marijuana, and cigarettes. They spoke in a rude, aggressive, and menacing way, projecting fear. I considered them like delinquent teenagers. I called in God/Source light, the spirits were sent to the light and released from the client's body. The client told me two days later that he had, had no further cigarettes or mood-altering substances.

We did a follow-up session on managing stress, anxiety, as the client had a lot of changes going on. We cleared childhood experiences and past life trauma.

On follow-up two weeks and six weeks later Shaun was still not smoking or using any substances.

These are just some of the many spirit releases that I've done throughout my work with clients, the physical, mental, emotional, and spiritual issues are often relieved or resolved simply by clearing the attached energy.

It is important to understand that in many cases (not all) the attached spirit is serving the client in some way. To release the spirit, we discover the reason the spirit is attached, and how, and clear any entanglements or anything that leaves the client open to attachments.

I teach my clients and students a variety of ways to clear attachments using theta healing, mediumship, access consciousness. it's also important to develop a relationship with yourself, your body, and your emotions so that you can discern the difference between yourself and others' energies, whether incarnate or discarnate. This is often such a difficult issue for empaths, spiritually inclined people, and people who have experienced a lot of trauma, who have very open energetic boundaries.

Daily energetic grounding is a wonderful way to keep your personal energy field clear and maintain your personal and energetic sovereignty. You'll find access to my meditations when you sign up for the book bonuses.

Spirit Release & Journey to the Golden City

In this session, my client was keen to connect with a past life. However, she found difficulty connecting with her Higher Self and questioned if there was a spirit attached to her. We ended up doing a spirit release, some inner child work, before going into the other lifetime, which turned out to be a very interesting experience.

SR: Something feels familiar from a dream I've had. As every night I've gone up to meditate, there's this dark figure that's kind of hanging on, and it feels male. Remembering my dream, it was this male that was trying to shut out an aspect obviously or maybe it's not mine; I don't know. But also, I'm going up, and I'm starting to see gold.

KL: Right. So, tell me a little bit more about this dark figure that's male. What does his energy feel like to you?

SR: Heavy, trying to hold me back. It's like I want to let go of his fingers in the cloud.

KL: So, his fingers are on the cloud?

SR: Yes, his fingers are on the cloud, and it's like he's trying to pull it down, or maybe I imagine it.

KL: So, let's find out, what's happening here. Does he have a name? Let's talk to him and see if maybe he has a message for you.

SR: I'm lost, so maybe that's the name?

KL: So, tell me, where are you lost?

SR: In the ethers, I don't have a home.

KL: For how long have you been lost?

SR: I'm hearing centuries and then light-years.

KL: How long have you been with Sally?

SR: I got too long, but I don't know whether that's him or me. I feel like I want to ask him where have you come from or are you a part of me.

KL: Have a look and see if there's a face.

SR: I don't see clearly; I just have a sense. I felt quite cold in my legs as I was going up.

KL: Yes, so maybe ask him.

SR: You think I am part of you. I'm not sure about this. My mind goes, am I?

KL: Okay, so let's just allow your mind to relax and let's allow your higher self to shine a light on this shadowy figure. And let's see who or what this shadowy figure is all about.

SR: I'm here to find a home.

KL: So, where have you come from?

SR: He doesn't know. I'm scratching my neck on the right.

KL: So, is this being creating the scratch in your neck?

SR: No.

KL: Are you connected to this being through any time/space dimensional reality? Why is he attached to you? Is there a connection, or is it just like a random cling on? What does he say?

SR: It's around my hip, more I can feel.

KL: Okay. Do you have a contract with him?

SR: No, I'm getting heat coming up as I'm connecting.

L: What does this being want? Does he know? Can we speak directly to him? What is it that you want? Are you aware that you don't have a body?

SR: No. I don't have a body.

KL: Would you like a body?

SR: I don't know, I just want to find home.

KL: And you don't know where home is?

SR: Not really. (The client's conscious mind comes in) I don't know whether it should be part of me. Have I ignored it?

KL: So, truth, is it a part of you?

SR: Okay, no, it's been around a long time, but I'm getting it's not a part of me.

KL: So, it's been around a long time, but it's not part of you. Allow yourself to relax and allow your conscious mind to step aside and your unconscious mind to guide you and support you. I'd like to speak directly to this being. Do you wish to go to the light, and from there, you will be able to go home, wherever home is?

SR: What does home feel like?

KL: You don't know what home feels like. How did you come to connect with Sally?

SR: She's happy to help.

KL: When did you first connect with Sally? Was it in this lifetime? Yeah, how old was she? (Four) Four I see, so what was going on at that time that drew you to her?

SR: She was looking for a companion. She was lost too.

KL: So, you came along? And you've been there ever since?

SR: I filled a hole.

KL: Yeah. So, do you have a name?

SR: Jai.

KL: Hello, Jai, would you like to speak to Sally, or would you like to go to the light?

SR: Why can't I stay here?

KL: Does it feel like home, where you are now?

SR: Not really.

KL: Do you have a family?

SR: I was abandoned.

KL: Why were you abandoned, Jai?

SR: I didn't conform.

KL: In what way?

SR: I didn't follow the rules.

KL: Oh. How old were you when you were abandoned and when you connected with Sally?

SR: I don't know. I'm hundreds of years old now. Well, I don't know, really.

KL: So, can you describe your body? Do you have a light body? Do you have a form? If we could give you what you want, what would it be?

SR: Well, I want to be loved, but I don't know what that feels like. Cos, I'm lost, and I don't know who I am or where I belong.

KL: Would you like to find out?

SR: Yeah.

KL: Tell me about your connection with Sally. Do you feel loved by Sally?

SR: Sometimes, she's nice to be around; she's like a friend. She's lost as well.

KL: Yeah. It's good to have friends. So, I wonder if you'd like to have friends without having to be lost. What if you could be happy? What if you could be free to have friends, be loved and be at home? Does that sound like something you'd like?

SR: Yes.

KL: And is there anybody that you know that you remember that you would like to see again?

SR: There is a father figure I can see.

KL: Oh, that's good.

SR: I have a vague image?

KL: And are you connected with him now?

SR: No, it was a long time ago.

KL: So, would you like to call him in? Just invite this father figure to come and be with you.

SR: He may not want to be with me.

KL: I'm sure that he will.

SR: I can't work out what he's wearing; he's light, quite muscular. He's got a spear and something over his head.

KL: What colour of skin has he got?

SR: Quite pale.

KL: How does he connect with Jai?

SR: He's holding his hand down.

KL: How does Jai feel?

SR: He's just kind of taking his hand and jumping onto him.

KL: He obviously trusts him then. So, I'm wondering whether Jai has any of your soul fragments and whether you have any of Jai's soul fragments?

SR: He's got some of mine.

KL: So, would Jai be willing to return your soul fragments?

SR: Yeah, he's kind of… he feels like he's throwing them.

KL: So, let's make sure that you have back all your soul fragments from Jai, washed and cleansed and integrated in the highest and best way possible. All Jai's soul fragments, be given back to him, washed and cleansed, so that you can both be whole and free now. What's happening now?

SR: Okay. Oh, he's going into the light. He's kind of looking back. It's kind of being willing to let him go too.

KL: Yeah, how are you feeling?

SR: There's warmth coming into my hip. I was going to say more complete but not quite.

KL: I wonder if there's a younger part of you that's present?

SR: Yeah, that was when I got emotional. When you connected with the child.

KL: So, is little Sally there? How does she feel about Jai going?

SR: A bit frightened, cos she's always had him as her friend, when she was lonely, someone who felt like her.

KL: What does she need right now?

SR: Just feeling her coming into my heart a bit more.

KL: I'm curious, does she have any of Jai's soul fragments, or does Jai have any of her soul fragments?

SR: I'm just checking. I'm getting no, but I'm aware my hip still feels a bit cool in one part. Ah, something's just coming from him. It feels like Joy.

KL: Ah, welcome the joy.

SR: So that feels complete; she is happy and joyful now.

KL: So, how does Jai feel? Is he happy with his father figure?

SR: Yes, he seems to be clinging on to him. Oh, they're ready to go now.

KL: Yeah. And how is little Sally feeling? Is she happy for Jai to go?

SR: She's waving now. Yeah.

KL: We can have lots of friends, can't we? As many friends as you like, or as few as you like. So, let's just wave goodbye to Jai and his father figure, so they can go home, wherever that may be.

SR: They just zoomed off.

KL: Oh, I wonder if little Sally might like to come on this journey as well, to travel in the cloud with you.

SR: She's alright; she's playing with Joy.

KL: She's happy; that's good. Okay, do you have an inner mother that you connect with?

SR: I haven't, really. I don't consciously connect with an inner mother.

KL: Yeah. So, I'm wondering, would little Sally like an inner mother? An inner mother is a great resource for nurturing and mothering us and supporting us, and they can be amazing Inner children but also for us as adults. So, my inner mother is Mother Mary; she came to me.

SR: Yeah. I have Mother Mary.

KL: Maybe you might introduce her to Mother Mary at some point.

SR: Yeah, they're together now.

(Having cleared the spirit attachment, we were now able to move forward with the regression.)

KL: Okay. So, do you want to continue on the cloud?

SR: Ah, I've been told there's a Golden City.

KL: Who's telling you about the Golden City, do you know?

SR: I don't know; it's just my Higher Self.

KL: So, just relax and know that you're free now to go to the Golden City. Let's go see what the Golden City is all about. Just allow your breath to take you deeper and deeper as you journey now on the cloud. When the cloud stops, you find yourself in the Golden City and tell me now, all that you see, hear, feel, and experience.

SR: I think I've been here before. I'm seeing lots of books and like an altar or stepping up on some level. I see books on the left, but I don't see anything on the right. I've never really looked on the right. If I look out, I feel a bit shivery actually, I don't know if that's the energies. It looks like this city I'm seeing. It's got purple and lights, and it's just (yawns) it's got lots of… I can't really see it, but it's got coloured lights.

KL: What colours are they?

SR: Purples and pinks and lilacs and, it's obviously a city, all I'm getting is a city, it's obviously, a higher-level city.

KL: Is it a Golden City?

SR: I'm not seeing gold so much, although there's a lot of light; it makes my eyes flicker. Apparently, just by thinking, I can go wherever I want. I've just heard I'm in the right place. Yeah. That came up. So, it's a bit like I'm feeling the energy of the city up through my body. Yeah.

KL: How does it feel?

SR: It's just like I'm clearing stuff at the moment. It's not home, but it's a place I often visit in my dream.

KL: Does this place have a name? Ask that energy that's coming up. Like, just get a sense of your connection, and what's available here.

SR: I just got Pleiades.

KL: I'm curious about these books you mentioned. Is there anything there for you?

SR: I'm seeing a gold cup, so I don't know whether I pulled out one, but I'm seeing a gold cup. (yawns) It's been filled up, with a jug, but I can't see who's pouring it. It looks like water. But this water is exceptionally clear. It's like programmed water if that makes sense. It's got information and codes in it, and then I'm meant to drink it.

KL: So, do you know what information and codes?

SR: Egypt, I'm getting, pyramids. I'm walking in the lands of the pharaohs, a time when I was there. I see a diamond in the desert sand, and I'm retrieving it. I'm in the King's chamber, and I'm aligning to the stars, I'm in the sarcophagus.

KL: Which stars are you aligning to?

SR: Sirius, I got Dog Star which is Sirius. There are others as well, and it's coming into that diamond.

KL: Are you holding the diamond?

SR: It's in my heart, and I'm realigning and holding the diamond. I'm stepping out; I'm taking it somewhere else now. I'm getting a sense of the original, the first pyramid or something.

KL: I wonder if you get a sense of a name that's you in Egypt in the pyramids.

SR: No. I feel I need to connect with that pyramid.

KL: Yeah. Can you get a sense of your body? Can you see if you're male or female?

SR: I'm male. I think.

KL: Can you get a sense of your role at that time?

SR: Yes, downloading and retrieving.

KL: I'm curious about you being in the pyramid. Is anybody allowed in the pyramid, or do you have to be of a certain rank?

SR: No, you must have a rank. That was my role, to download the information from the stars. So, I'm in that first pyramid, there is something there I need to do or take back with me. It's quite dark in there. I'm just feeling my way along the wall with my hands.

KL: Does that enable you to know where you're going?

SR: I saw a dagger, and then I thought perhaps it's an Ankh. I'm not sure.

KL: So, there's a little difference between those two (laughing).

SR: Both are gold.

KL: So, is it one or the other, or both?

SR: I think it could be both actually. I can see the dagger going in my right hip, down my leg, as if it's got a holder, but it's got rubies in the cross point; it's a small one.

KL: Ah, so it's not going in your hip; it's just going down your leg?

SR: Yeah.

KL: That's good to clarify. (laughing)

SR: (Laughs) Yes, it was quite an ornamental one, if you know what I mean.

KL: What is the significance of the dagger?

SR: I'm getting status and protection. It was something I left behind. The Ankh is golden, hmm, interesting… I'm wondering whether it's going over my head or as a necklace, pendant, but as my words come out, it's going over my head?

KL: Yes, it's going over your head and then what happens?

SR: I feel a bit of pain in my shoulders, in my collarbone, so maybe it's like healing.

KL: You say it's like a necklace that's gone over your head. How is your collarbone feeling now?

SR: Yeah, it's passed, the ankh is going into the sand, the energy of it. Now I can come out of the pyramid, and I'm out in the Sphinx now. Getting around the top between the paws. I'm giving thanks. It seems like I'm meditating, and the sun is rising behind. Now, I'm underneath, walking in the halls.

KL: Do these halls have a name?

SR: I'm not sure; I'm not getting one.

KL: Ok, so what's in the halls?

SR: I've been here before, and I can see the Ark of The Covenant again. Thoth is there, and Anubis and Isis.

KL: Almost a full house!

SR: Isis is standing in front of me. I think she's doing something, but I'm not quite sure what. For a moment, it was like I was seeing all the people I'd been.

KL: What did you see?

SR: I don't know; it was just a sense, flashing faces, priestess, queen, all the different people I've been. (yawns)

I feel like I'm going down, and then I'm saying dolphins, so it's like I'm in the sea.

I'm not quite sure why I'm here, really.

KL: So, are you swimming with the dolphins in the water?

SR: Yeah, I went a bit floaty, actually,

KL: Yeah, so are you in the sea, or are you somewhere else?

SR: Yes, I'm deep in the sea, clear good things.

KL: Yes, sometimes it's good to float and allow the water to support you. How does your body feel?

SR: Feels at home, actually. Don't have to do much; I can just be.

KL: I wonder if you might like to anchor that feeling in your body? Floating, relaxing, nothing to do, just being and feeling at home.

SR: I'm with the dolphins; they're swimming next to me, not holding me but supporting me.

KL: Do the dolphins have a message for you?

SR: They're always here and a reminder of freedom and play and joy. I'm just feeling that there. I can hear them squeaking and talking. Oh, just feeling that playful energy, feeling it rather than hearing anything.

KL: Yeah. So, let's just anchor those energies in your body, into every cell of your being, every atom, every molecule, freedom, play, joy, relaxation.

SR: Okay, I'm getting I've got all the wisdom of the ages within me. I just need to flow with that. I don't have to prove myself.

(Long silence)

SR: I'm being shown this diamond again. No, it's not. It's made of diamond, but it's a star with five or six points. It's in the centre, that's what I see that I am.

SR: Maybe it's my Merkabah I see.

KL: Why don't you ask the star. Twinkle, twinkle, little star.

SR: Yeah, it's the essence of who I am.

KL: I'm hearing it's not so little either.

SR: I feel quite warm now. I was just asking what does my star want for me? I just got for me to be whole.

KL: What's required for you to be whole?

SR: I get expanding into the wholeness of who I am. Now, I'm seeing lots of bright lights. So, although I can still feel my body, I can feel like my light has expanded. Yeah, I feel quite expanded to me

KL: Beautiful, so I'm curious why your higher self has bought you here and if there's anything your higher self wants to share with you at this time?

SR: Recognising myself as light and recognising my worth and all that I've done. Now that I know that I can be all that I am is what I'm hearing.

KL: So, are you home now?

SR: Yeah. I feel that in my heart.

KL: Yeah, beautiful. Is there anything else your higher self wants to share?

SR: Keep feeding the light within, keep seeing my light and not looking for a reason to clear.

KL: Yeah.

SR: Not looking for areas to clear, just being this light. I'm seeing that's all I need do, it sounds simple. I'm told to keep accepting my worth.

KL: How do you feel about accepting your worth?

SR: I'm getting weight in gold.

KL: Worth your weight in gold. Yeah.

SR: Yeah. Just taking that in a bit. I can feel it in my upper heart.

KL: What's the energy that you feel?

SR: Love, recognition, gratitude as well.

KL: Wonderful. I wonder if your highest self has anything to share about your relationship with Michael or your business.

SR: I'm getting things are changing. The magic is already woven. I'm just seeing threads of gold that have been threaded between us, so it's being patient. Remember to come from love. It's kind of accepting what I see in him. Not to take any of his comments personally; it's just what he's going through. When I love myself completely, then I can accept him completely, and then any comments are kind of deflected or bounce off, and I can choose to see through that and see the illusion but see through that.

KL: That sounds like great advice from your higher self.

SR: Yeah. I'm getting, like, trust in myself and really trusting my intuition and wisdom deeply, all much deeper than I had before. It's okay to follow my path. You've chosen a very kind of independent way of moving through your life, so don't feel you're not keeping up or not doing what other people are doing. It's all society's conditioning.

KL: So, don't compare yourself, don't worry. Yeah

SR: All in good time. Yes, disciplined approach but not dogmatic. Allowing the energy to flow when it's there and when it's not, that's okay. Trust that. In terms of the publisher because I've started conversations, my heart already knows.

KL: What is it you already know? Do you know what you already know?

SR: Well, my heart knows what I want, what is acceptable and who I will work with. Maybe my mind and heart haven't truly… I'll just ask whether I've met them or not.

Okay, I get no. I'm not sure about that. So, I need a bit of time. And maybe that's an unreasonable question.

KL: Hmm. Is there anything that you need to know or for your heart and your mind to be aligned? Or is it just a case of time?

SR: I think it's my mind must align more with my heart.

KL: And I wonder if your subconscious can align your heart and your mind now.

SR: It feels like my mind has gone very quiet; it feels like I'm just sitting and being in my heart. I don't need to decide yet; it will all become clear.

KL: Beautiful, yes, everything is in divine timing.

Reflections

This was a beautiful session, we hadn't expected to be doing a spirit release, but that led to a beautiful healing. The client suffers with diabetes, which is often linked to a lack of joy, so it was wonderful for the client to reconnect with her inner child and her joy and to retrieve past life gifts, abilities and receive guidance from her higher self, regarding her relationship and her work.

Hypnosis is a wonderful way to connect with both the subconscious (lower unconscious) and the superconscious (higher mind) and enables wonderful healing processes to take place on all levels of mind, body, and spirit. When working with clients with current life issues I may connect the client with inner resources such as the inner child, higher self, inner mother, inner father, inner mate, subpersonalities, loved ones in spirit, spirit guides, ascended masters. When doing past life regression, the higher self and/or spirit guides, or galactic beings are often the most useful resources available.

Healing in this way may include

- Scanning and identifying physical, mental, emotional, and spiritual roots of illness and disease.
- Releasing negative or toxic energies, spirit attachments.
- Receiving physical, mental, emotional, and spiritual healing.
- Receiving healing insights, remedies, elixirs.
- Receive healing and light-body activations from spirit or galactic beings.

Many times, the client is taken to a wonderful healing place, such as a special cave, a healing lake, a waterfall, or in the case of galactic assistance, sometimes the client may be taken to a healing pod, where they receive sound and light technology healing. I have been given elixirs and flower remedies by my inner healer on occasion and received many light activations and healing from spirit guides and galactic beings as they work energetically with root cause of issues, be that in mind, body, or spirit.

Many years back when I was training in hypnotherapy, in a hypnosis demonstration on another student, I saw a gentleman whose legs were paralysed and who was using a wheelchair as he couldn't walk unaided. In trance when he was invited to speak with his legs, he expressed anger and was invited to kick and push with his legs. (I and other students on the training were sat around with cushions that he was pushing his legs against.) We were all amazed to see the power, movement, and strength in his legs as he pushed and kicked against the cushions, expressing his anger and frustration. Later out of the trance he was unable to move his legs.) On a soul level, everything in life is serving us in some way, and we are learning lessons, and experiencing challenges that support our souls' growth and evolution. Often our body carries cellular memory of traumas whether in this life or past lives, which have been carried forward or imprinting from the ancestral level or soul level. When we work with the subconscious and higher self, we can gain an understanding of these lessons and heal mind, body, and spirit.

Our bodies are pretty magical and are governed by our unconscious mind. Many times, when working with clients as a medical intuitive, their body speaks to me and I am shown various organs or parts of the body that are holding memories and emotions, and beliefs. Once these memories, energies, and beliefs are released, the client gains improvement on physical, mental, emotional, and spiritual levels. As a full-body empath and medical intuitive and body whisperer, I'm blessed to be able to support my clients in their healing process. This is a process that I also teach my students. In hypnosis, the higher self and the inner healer can help the client to commune with their body. This is a wonderful gift.

Note: Hypnosis and energy healing are not a substitute for medical care and clients are always advised to consult their doctor. Many times, the healing received from the client's higher self and spirit can and does relieve physical symptoms and it can also be used as an adjunct to medical care to support the client's healing process.

Cyril The Ovarian Cyst

The following client-therapist dialogue was transcribed from a live somatic healing hypnotherapy session that was recorded on video. It demonstrates the wide variety of processes that are combined within transpersonal hypnotherapy and advanced somatic healing. You will see elements of emotional clearing, inner guide work, subpersonalities, attachments and spirit release, past life regression, and somatic healing all woven seamlessly into the session. In these types of sessions, the client's higher self, inner healer, or spirit guide scans the body.

Due to the confidential nature of this material, there were times I gave the client permission to process silently, so you may experience gaps in your comprehension of the dialogue. As a therapist, it is important not to get hooked on the client's story but to allow cathartic release and resolution of the presenting issue. In this session, the client was able to gain insight, release negative thoughts and feelings, and anchor positive resources within her body.

KL: All right, Charlotte. So, would you like to say a little bit about what you would like to work with today?

CB: Yeah, I've been recently diagnosed with a rather large ovarian cyst. The doctor said that he feels I've had it for several years. However, since Christmas, I've noticed a rather large abdominal swelling, where the cyst has made a lot of progress in the last three months. So, I'm here to basically focus on the cyst and see what's going on in there.

(Note the client was under medical supervision with her doctor and was booked for surgery just two weeks later.)

KL: Okay. Great. I understand you've named your cyst.

CB: I have indeed. Cyril. Cyril the cyst.

KL: Cyril the Cyst. That's an interesting name! So, it's going to be interesting to talk with Cyril and find out what's happening.

CB: Yeah. Absolutely!

KL: Okay. Fantastic! So, I want you to make yourself comfortable.

I take the client into trance, connecting her with her inner child, her inner mother, inner healer, and higher self.

CB: (Deep breath) I've got ripping flesh, with lots of red. It's like tearing meat from bones. Red meat. All I can see are these teeth and this mouth. I can see this ball and like a head coming out of the ball with teeth. It's like the cyst is what I can see.

KL: So just take a nice deep breath knowing that you're safe, just allowing yourself to relax as these images become clearer and clearer to you now. It's as though you're watching a movie screen, and you can pause or fast forward or rewind whenever you need. What's happening now?

CB: (Deep sigh) I'm in this… there are loads of trees and like undergrowth around me, and I've got a slab and just chopping, chopping bones. Chopping.

KL: Who is chopping bones? (Links with previous past life session where the client chopped up babies as part of a sacrificial ritual)

CB: Feels like me, but it's not me. I'm male.

KL: So, you're chopping bones, and you're male. And who else is there? Take a moment to look around and notice who else is there.

CB: It's just animals around me.

KL: Animals. Uh-huh.

CB: Like a wild hog and boar, running around, a dog, bones and…

KL: So, you're outside?

CB: Mm-hmm.

KL: Tell us about these bones that you're chopping. Where are the bones coming from?

CB: It looks like chickens—small chickens. (Client becomes distressed.) It's more than that.

KL: As the client was distressed, I used some dissociation so she could be more comfortable. Sometimes cathartic release is useful and a part of the healing process and equally I don't want to re-traumatise my client. Take a nice, deep relaxing breath and just rely on yourself to accept whatever appears on the screen, just like a movie. Nice deep breath. Just relax. As though you're watching a movie. And as you watch that movie up there on the screen, you can see everything that's happening. And you don't have to be attached to the feelings. It's just a movie. Allow yourself to relax.

CB: (Sobbing)

KL: What's happening now?

CB: I can't even say.

KL: Okay. Just take a nice deep breath and know that whatever is going on right now, whatever it is that you can't even say, it's not happening now. It's in the past, and you're viewing it now on this movie screen. That's it, take a nice deep breath. Knowing that you're safe, that you can trust your unconscious mind and your inner healer, your body's own natural wisdom, to guide you today as you begin to understand and explore the healing of Cyril. I wonder if you'd like to speak to Cyril right now. Have you spoken to Cyril before?

CB: Not really.

KL: So just taking a moment to focus on your body, calling in your inner healer to be with you, giving you wisdom and strength. Is there anybody else you'd like to call in to be with you now to help you? Who would you like to call in?

CB: My inner mother.

KL: So, call in your inner mother to be with you now to guide you. What would you like to say to Cyril?

CB: I'm sorry.

KL: You're sorry? What are you sorry for?

CB: For what I've done.

KL: What did you do? Is this the 'something' that you don't want to say?

CB: (Client is crying) I didn't know what I was doing when I had done it. I didn't know what I was doing.

KL: It's okay. So, you're sorry, and you didn't know what you were doing.

CB: No. I didn't know how it would feel until after.

KL: And how did it feel after? Can you tell Cyril?

CB: Really bad. Really, really, really bad. I've done it before. I've done it now, and I've done it before.

(Client is talking here about past life actions and a termination she had in her current life, which she regrets.)

KL: But you didn't know? What does Cyril say? Can you be aware of Cyril now?

CB: Yeah, Cyril is weak.

KL: Weak? What do you mean weak?

CB: (long pause) Cyril feels like (sighs) guilt. Cyril feels weak right now.

KL: And I wonder if we could speak directly to Cyril right now. Can you see Cyril? Just taking a nice deep breath, allowing yourself to become aware of Cyril now in some way. Perhaps you're even becoming Cyril right now. That's it. Hi, Cyril.

CB: (Moans quietly)

KL: How are you? You know we're here today to speak with you and find out what you need and help you. Would you be willing to talk to me today?

CB: (Moans quietly)

KL: That's great. And how do you feel about Charlotte?

CB: I'm angry and sad.

KL: You're angry with Charlotte, and you feel sad.

CB: Frustrated.

KL: *Well, it sounds as though Charlotte has done something quite bad that she regrets that she doesn't really want to talk about. What do you want?*

CB: Kindness.

KL: Kindness. Are you a part of Charlotte? So, you want some kindness. And what would that look like to you, Cyril? What would that kindness look like or feel like or sound like?

CB: Inner peace.

KL: Yeah. And are you able to tell us when you were created? When you came into being? How long have you been with Charlotte?

CB: Since the birth of her first child.

KL: The birth of her first child, okay. Were you around before that?

CB: Yeah.

KL: Okay. Charlotte said that you felt as though you were her guilt, is that right?

CB: I am.

KL: So, do you like affecting Charlotte in this way? You're in her stomach right now and causing a bit of a problem, aren't you? And do you know that the surgeons want to cut you out?

CB: I know.

KL: And what you'd really like is to be shown a little bit of kindness and love and some peace. Would you like to see Charlotte healthy, feeling good and happy?

CB: Hmm.

KL: So, what is it that needs to happen? What does Charlotte need to do right now to set you free? To release this guilt and shame?

CB: Stop being so angry with herself.

KL: Okay. And how can Charlotte stop feeling angry with herself as that is obviously something that Charlotte did quite a long time ago? Are we talking about this lifetime?

CB: This lifetime and one before.

KL: And I wanted to know if it's possible for us to go back in time now. What do you need to show Charlotte? Those people that she hurt, even though she didn't know at the time, and she maybe wasn't fully aware or conscious of exactly what was happening. So, calling in her higher self now to shed light and illumination for all those situations that took place to begin to understand the bigger picture. To see any contracts in place with those particular people and the soul lessons and what you were learning from them. Calling those people forward now and asking for forgiveness, speaking from your heart, letting them know how much sorrow, how much shame, how much guilt you've carried through all this time.

CB: So much shame.

KL: That's right. So much shame. So, as we connect with those people now looking into their eyes, feeling into their soul, your heart open, what happens now?

CB: I feel love.

KL: You feel love? Where does that love come from?

CB: I don't know why these people are standing around me.

KL: Who is standing around you? Are they people you know?

CB: I've got an angel with wings.

KL: Do you know her name?

CB: It's actually… it's my inner mother with wings.

KL: Oh, how wonderful.

CB: She's trying to give me something, but I can't see what it is. It's like a wand.

KL: Now, take a nice deep breath. Allow yourself to relax. So just allow your inner mother now to give you guidance. How can you use that wand? What it's for?

CB: It's a crystal ball.

KL: Fantastic. What does she want you to do with this crystal ball?

CB: She's holding it up to the light. She's telling me to look up. Look up into the light.

KL: That's right, so just take a nice deep breath and look up into the light.

CB: There's peace in there.

KL: What's happening now?

CB: (Sobbing) She's showing me forgiveness. I see a rainbow. It's like I'm sitting in the dark, and she's showing me the light. I've got a cloak of shame and a cloak of guilt.

KL: What would need to happen now for you to let go of those cloaks? Take them off once and for all.

CB: Dirty, dark, and sticky. I stink.

KL: Would you like to ask those people if it's okay for you to take those cloaks off?

CB: Yeah, I'd like to see them gone.

KL: So, they're not angry, they're not sad about what happened?

CB: The people that I hurt are very angry inside. They never asked for it. They had no choice, and I had no choice. What's done is done. I have done what I was told to do.

KL: What were the lessons that you learned from this situation?

CB: Question things before you do them. Don't just do as you're told. Don't just follow somebody's lead.

KL: That's a very powerful lesson to learn, isn't it? To just stand in your own power and perhaps connect with your own heart and see what feels right for you. So, what would need to happen for you to let go of this cloak of shame and guilt and perhaps for those people to let go of their anger and sadness and to gain understanding from their higher selves? Perhaps the soul lessons that were learned by all of you as we come into this life and go through experiences. Perhaps we don't understand on the conscious level, but there's always a purpose on the soul level. I'm sure you've learned powerful lessons, I'm sure that they too have learned lessons.

CB: I've got like… I'm trying to take off the shame and guilt, but I feel like I need to hold onto it. I need to keep it with me. Like I have to protect it. Love it, nurture it.

KL: So, would you take a moment now and just allow yourself to go deeper and deeper into your body. Deeper and deeper into Cyril. Connect with that part you want to hold on to and nurture. Just allow yourself to go deeper and deeper into that part that you want to nurture and tell me what you experience. You don't want to let go. You really want to keep holding on to it.

CB: It's part of me.

KL: Just allow yourself to become more aware of that part of you. What does it look like?

CB: It's horrible. It's dirty.

KL: Does it have a form?

CB: It's hairy with teeth.

KL: And you don't like it? But at the same time, you feel that you want to nurture it.

CB: I want to protect it. I want to hold on to it too.

KL: Just allow your unconscious mind, your inner mother, and your inner healer to guide you and support you on this journey. These wonderful healing journeys. As we go back there to the time when this part of you was first created. Tell me what you experience.

CB: I'm on holiday with my parents, my husband, and my little girl.

KL: What is happening?

CB: We played on the lawn outside where we were staying.

KL: What happens next?

CB: There's a holiday where I'm with my family and my mum is there.

KL: Your mum's there with you?

CB: My mum, my dad, and my mum's friends. Hayley is about three months old.

KL: And what happens? And so now you just have to see how this part of you was created. This part that you want to reject – the hairy thing with teeth. You want to reject it, but also you want to nurture it. How did it come into being?

CB: There's a connection there with my mother.

KL: What's the connection? Do you understand the connection?

CB: It's like my daughter gave my mother a mothering role, nurturing.

KL: I wonder if it's possible to speak to that hairy thing with teeth right now. Does it have a name? What's it called?

CB: The hairy thing with teeth is Cyril.

KL: Okay, so can we speak to Cyril? Cyril, I wonder if you can tell us more about how you came into being.

CB: Around this time, Charlotte was on holiday with her mum and dad and friend and her husband and a little girl.

KL: And that's when you first came into being? Are you a part of Charlotte? And is there any part of you, Cyril, which isn't a part of Charlotte?

CB: There's a part that's her mother that she doesn't like.

KL: So, I wonder if it's possible, Cyril, for you to let go of that part that's not you, not Charlotte. That part that Charlotte doesn't like. Would you like to let go of that part?

CB: Yeah.

KL: So, let's invite your inner mother and your inner healer and your higher self to give you an understanding of how this part came into being. It's not a part of you.

CB: It's an angry part.

KL: Mm-hmm. Are you able to let that part go? Are you able to release that part so that it can heal?

CB: Mm-hmm.

KL: So just allow your inner mother and your higher self to guide you now as you heal and release that part. Perhaps, understanding why, in some way, you invited that part to be with you. Perhaps, it served a purpose. Allowing yourself to now receive all of the learnings you need to release this part and allow it to heal, at the same time healing yourself, healing Cyril. What's happening now?

CB: I'm aware of all the anger and frustration that built up. I feel that part that was given to me by my mother. Again, not questioning it, just doing it. Repeating it and being what I was shown then – being angry with others when I needn't have been. I could have been more understanding.

KL: What was the positive purpose of that part? What did that part provide you with? Being angry with people? What did that give you?

CB: Power.

KL: So perhaps there was a lesson there in learning to be within your own power. Is there anything else you need to learn about empowering yourself and empowering others?

CB: Learning to say no.

KL: So perhaps you can say no right now to that part, thanking it for all that is shared with you, giving you a very powerful lesson to have learned. You can release it now that you understand the lesson. Is there anything you'd like to say to your mum?

CB: No. Not right now. It's not a very nice thing, I can't tell her what I want to say.

KL: So why don't you ask your inner mother if she can help you with that? Where in your body do you feel that is not a very nice thing that you want to say?

CB: In Cyril.

KL: And as you focus on that feeling, still allowing your inner mother to help you and just gently release those feelings. Whatever they are, all those feelings that your body has held on to, those feelings have been unexpressed. Those feelings need to be expressed and released now—your inner mother, your inner healer guiding you. See your mother before you, perhaps telling her all the things you'd like to have said to her.

CB: I want to smack her face in.

KL: You feel really angry.

CB: I've got tension in my jaw. The teeth are coming back; there's stress.

KL: There are those teeth. What do those teeth want to say?

CB: (Clicking her teeth together) It just goes argh (mumbling).

KL: I wonder if there's something else there with those teeth, another feeling?

CB: Yeah. So tight in my jaw.

KL: Is this the thing that you wanted to hold on to and nurture?

CB: I don't want to hold onto that, but it's a part of me. I want to hold onto me.

KL: Not now. It's not a part of you.

CB: It's as if I want it to be a part of me, it's part of me, but I don't want it to be a part of me. But if I let go, I'll lose my power; that's what it feels like.

KL: So, in a sense, it's a part of you that protects you.

CB: Mm-hmm. It keeps me safe.

KL: And I wonder if there is another way that you can be powerful and safe. Learn to say no. Learn to think for yourself rather than doing everything you're told. I wonder if there's another way you can learn to speak up for yourself and express your thoughts and your feelings.

CB: In a way, which doesn't hurt like this.

KL: Is that possible?

CB: I believe so.

KL: Is that possible right now?

CB: Yeah. If I ask for help more.

KL: And who are you going to ask?

CB: My inner mother. My inner healer.

KL: So, I want you to take your attention back to your belly and back to Cyril. What's happened to the hairy thing with teeth?

CB: It got smaller. It shrunk.

KL: It shrunk? Fantastic. And how do you feel about it now?

CB: Ok. I don't feel so tight.

KL: It's just a feeling, isn't it? A feeling of wanting to fight back. Maybe you wanted to protect yourself. Feeling angry and hurt, and you've learned that you can be assertive when you feel angry or hurt. You can protect yourself, put a boundary, and express your thoughts and feelings, and you don't need to hurt other people.

CB: I know.

KL: You can come from that place within you that's loved, that loves you, that loves others.

CB: In a loving way and not in a nasty way.

KL: And you know, sometimes, people do feel hurt, and they might have their own programs running, might take things in the wrong way. Wonder if your inner mother can help you in managing those situations so that you feel good within yourself and you can now act in a way that feels right to you, allowing yourself to release all anger, all guilt, all shame, releasing now any of those mother issues that don't belong to you; Releasing them now, thanking your mother for all that you've learned—perhaps seeing your mother now in a new light, knowing that she was also a product of her programming and conditioning. Can you feel the love between yourself and your mother?

CB: I've given her to the angels.

KL: And what's happening now?

CB: I've given her away, but there's a tie between us. There's like a cord between us.

KL: And do you need that cord?

CB: I do, and I don't.

KL: So, there's a part of you that needs that cord. Can we speak to that part of you that needs that cord right now? Just take a nice, deep, relaxing breath, becoming aware of that part of you that needs your mother, needs that cord, needs to feel attached.

CB: This kid is needy, wimpy, and whiny.

KL: How old is that part of you?

CB: Three.

KL: Three? Hello. So, we're speaking to little Charlotte.

CB: Mm-hmm. Clinging on to her mum's neck.

KL: Now, what would you like to say to little Charlotte right now? The little Charlotte that's still clinging on.

CB: Come with me. I can show you a different way; show you a new way.

KL: Is that what she needs to hear?

CB: She's not getting any attention, so there's no point staying there.

KL: Would you like to give Charlotte a big hug?

CB: Mm-hmm. (Giggles)

KL: As you hold her in your arms, giving her all the love and support that she needs from her mom, you and your inner mother feeling that wonderful, loving connection. Can you release your mother now?

CB: Yeah, yeah.

KL: She did her best, as most mothers do. How's little Charlotte feeling now?

CB: Acknowledged and safe.

KL: And is there anything that little Charlotte wants right now?

CB: Just lots of love, lots of understanding.

KL: So, I wonder if you'd like to put aside some time, maybe daily, to check in with little Charlotte and your inner mother. It's just time to play. You're always giving to other people. It's just time to give to yourself, to your inner child. So, as you continue to hold little Charlotte there, why don't you go back to your tummy and just become aware of what's happening in your tummy now.

CB: It feels tight. It feels like there is a lump.

KL: So why don't you take a nice deep breath. I'd like to speak to Cyril. I'd like Cyril to come forward.

CB: Cyril's a lot happier.

KL: A lot happier Cyril; that's good. I wonder if there's anything else that you need right now, Cyril?

CB: Be careful. Take care of her body.

KL: And what specifically would you like Charlotte to do? What does she need to do to look after her body?

CB: Nurture me in the way I was trying to nurture Cyril.

KL: That's right. You need to nurture yourself. Now that you've released that guilt and that shame, and you've forgiven yourself, I wonder if Cyril can help you. Perhaps, remind you and give you a nudge now and then. Like when you get too busy.

CB: He's smiling. The teeth are gone.

KL: So, the teeth are gone.

CB: Mm-hmm.

KL: Fantastic. I'd like to now invite your inner healer to connect with you and with Cyril. See if there's anything else that needs to take place; to heal the cyst that Cyril has created. Perhaps Cyril will be able to help you there.

CB: Drink more?

KL: Mm-hmm. That's a really good idea; when you're releasing, you need to drink more water. That's right. Clear out the toxins in your body. Fantastic. So, taking your hand and placing your hand on your body now, placing it over Cyril, allow yourself to love that part of you—a part of you that sometimes cares too much for other people and not enough for yourself. And as you've made that connection again with your inner child, that commitment to check in on a daily basis, to connect with your inner mother and your inner child, to allow Cyril to give you a nudge, perhaps when you forget; when you try to take on too much, Cyril will be able to just gently talk to you now, now that you're aware of his positive intention. You're aware that he's trying to protect you and nurture you. You're just allowing that cyst, allowing Cyril to receive all the love and gratitude; it's a wonderful lesson that he has shared with you as you begin to understand much more clearly now the lesson, allowing that energy to release through your body it's only energy. And now that the energy's purpose has become clear, you can allow it to just dissolve, take the learnings and knowledge insight, and those new behaviours forward now to a much healthier, happier life, knowing that your unconscious mind to begin right now to heal on a deeper level. Your inner healer, your inner mother, and Cyril, with your help, healing your body now, healing that cyst that begins to shrink and dissolve, flushing away and clearing all that energy. I wonder if Cyril has a colour.

CB: Purple.

KL: Purple. And Cyril, would you be happy to let this cyst go now? Are you happy that Charlotte understands why you've created that cyst? And of course since you're a part of Charlotte and the part that she needs to empower herself and let Charlotte inside. We don't want to get rid of you. Will you promise to help out Charlotte in the future? Help her live a happier, healthier life? Remind her when she needs reminding to look after herself? To rest?

CB: Yes.

KL: That's fantastic. Thank you, Cyril. And so allow Cyril and your inner mother and your inner healer to continue to work with you and your body, releasing the cyst easily and naturally with its own energy and as you allow that wonderful love that you are, that wonderful sense of compassion and understanding, to flow through every part of your body now, flowing into your ovaries, around your womb space, allowing your womb and your ovaries to release all that's no longer needed, just letting it go. See that energy flowing now and releasing through your body. What's happening now?

CB: It's feeling much softer now.

KL: Can you see and of that purple energy?

CB: It's gone pink and purple.

KL: As you continue to focus on that energy, knowing that it's only energy, allowing it to move through your body and maybe it wants to go up or down or around. Trusting your body, because your body knows what needs to happen to release this energy. So just allowing the energy to soften, flow and release. It's only energy. And with each and every breath you take, the energy of love, compassion, acceptance, forgiveness flows stronger and stronger within you now. Allowing each and every cell, every atom, every molecule, every organ in your body to be filled with love and light, feeling lighter and brighter with all the energy, with the last remnants continuing to release, knowing that you can connect with your body any time. Is there something else you want to say?

CB: I feel like it's here. (Puts her hand higher up on her body, indicating the energy is moving up and out)

KL: That's good. You're just allowing it to soften and flow, and you can use your hands to just guide the energy to release. It's only energy, allowing this energy to soften, flow and release. Good. That's it. Just releasing now. Good. All that tension, energy, old energy – just release it - the memories, releasing now. Good.

CB: (Burps) **(client releasing energy here.)**

KL: That's right. It's only energy. Allow your inner healer to take your hands to guide the energy and assist the energy to release. And your inner healer now bringing in the most wonderful healing light if you're using your body – a beautiful healing light, giving you warmth and love as you continue to release the old energy. That's it. Good. That's it. All that tension releasing. Oh, it's going to be a really cheap facelift.

CB: (Giggles)

KL: Yes, that's right. Good. Yeah. That's right. And just allow your face to fill with love from a gentle touch from your inner healer, soothing, smoothing, and healing. Maybe your inner healer can take you to the waterfall and stand just under the waterfall - allow that wonderful, natural, innocent energy of the waterfall to restore your sense of innocence and beauty.

(Healing ceremony/ritual to release shame and guilt. Direct suggestion to guide and reinforce positive changes.)

KL: So just feeling that water upon you – each tiny drop of water that splashes upon your body, recharging you, revitalizing you, bringing you back to love. Feel your energy softening, feel that wonderful sense of joy deep within you bubbling up with each and every breath, feeling more and more relaxed. More and more happy, safe, secure, loved, supported, innocent and free – free to be who you are, because who you are is so beautiful, so special. Feel yourself shining like a star in the sky. See the smile on people's faces, free to talk to them, just being yourself. And any time, you want to remember this feeling, you can do so easily and naturally, simply by placing your hand upon your body, perhaps when you try it, just as you are doing right now, you'll feel an incredible sense of love and joy as your body is sparkling with the truth of who you are. And the love and the light that is you is shining out for all to see and experience. See before you now a beautiful mirror, an endless mirror, a most magnificent light shining out. It's almost dazzling you, and you're so surprised, but this is who you are. You are that light that's reflecting from you now. That light and love is you, reflecting light and love to you, nurturing you, refreshing you. Notice how it feels in your body when you love yourself. So just continue to allow this love to flow through you, knowing that you can return and connect with your body, your higher self, your inner mother, your inner child, and Cyril is now lovingly supporting you in nurturing yourself and empowering yourself, thanking you for all the help and the love and support, remembering all the lessons and holding on to that wand and crystal ball from your inner mother. Just in your own time, bringing yourself back now into waking consciousness, becoming aware now of your body, aware of the couch, wiggling fingers and toes as you're coming back into waking consciousness, coming back into your body, feeling refreshed, feeling relaxed, getting ready to open your eyes and as you open them now, in 5, 4, 3, 2, 1 you're wide awake relaxed, refreshed and alert, remembering all that you need to remember now.

CB: Hello.

KL: Welcome back.

CB: Oh, my word.

KL: Well, that was a journey.

CB: Wasn't it? I was able to connect with everybody again.

KL: Yeah. How are you feeling now? How did that feel?

CB: Absolutely wonderful. I haven't been there for a while.

KL: Yeah. And so, it's important to use our resources when we make these connections. Then we can tap into our own inner resources and healing, which I already connected in some way with Cyril in the beginning to understand. You know there was more going on. Fantastic. Well done.

CB: (Giggles) Thank you. My word, that was amazing!

Note: This client had done some work with me prior to this session, so was familiar with the transpersonal hypnotherapy concepts and processes, so I found it easy to connect her very quickly with the established inner guides. Due to the confidential nature of the material and the fact that we were on film, I used my discretion to allow the client to process silently at times. At times, both she and I knew a deeper layer of what was happening, as she had previously done past life work that linked with this session.

Client's Reflection on Follow Up

'I'm very well, thank you. The operation went well, and I'm so much more comfortable now at last. The pressure no longer on my bladder is bliss. I've found since our session with Cyril that a weight has been lifted from my shoulders. I have felt a lot lighter in myself, plus now my cyst has gone, my energy has increased loads already. Friends and family have said how much better I look and are impressed by my strong upbeat attitude and manner!

I feel like I've turned a corner which has been a long time coming! We had a laugh when we got back to mine. David walked in from the garden and handed me a chicken wishbone that he had found. I couldn't believe it after the laugh we had, over the chickens, the chicken barbeque, and the laugh over the wishbones. David just stood there wondering what was so funny, which made it even funnier - bless him!

P.S. I got hold of a lovely chicken coup today, and the kids are going to paint it all the colours of a rainbow! Wicked...'

Synchronicity in action here confirms the work that the client has done on the etheric and causal plane. The client had for some time been talking of getting a few chickens, so the higher self is using the process of nurturing the chickens as a way of atonement here. Painting the chicken coup in the colours of the rainbow links with the rainbow that the client was shown by her inner mother. This was a wonderful result for the client, and I wonder what might have happened had she come earlier to work on this issue.

Afterword

We are living in challenging times, times of great change, when many of the 'usual' ways of doing things are not working, and radical change is needed, which includes the need for us all to acknowledge our shadow selves, to release our personal and collective traumas, relinquish old, outdated conditioning and subconscious programming, to connect with our divinity, embrace our true self, realise self-mastery, and claim our sovereignty. As we do this, we can embrace our destiny and evolution as divine beings, living in harmony with ourselves, one another, and our beautiful planet and thus create a more loving, joyful, and conscious world for all.

As we embody higher levels of consciousness, we will create solutions that will eliminate and eradicate many of the global issues we are currently facing such as poverty, climate change, economy, housing, social care, education, and crime to name a few.

This book has been written to awaken you to your own truth and I realise it may well leave some of you with many questions. I have my own understanding and experience of our soul's journey, and the changes that are currently taking place on earth, having recalled, or experienced in trance, meditation, channelling, shamanic journeys, hypnosis, and sometimes spontaneous past-life recall over the years and having now facilitated thousands of past life regressions. I believe the best way to learn is through personal experience, for it is our personal experience and journey that truly transforms us on all levels of mind, body, spirit, allowing us to embrace and embody our divinity, thus creating heaven on earth.

My invitation is for you to reflect and ponder on your own soul journey and if you feel called, to explore your own soul's journey, your soul's origin, your soul's purpose, to heal any shadow or trauma, to explore all that is possible for you, so that you can shine bright, live in joy and peace, and live a rich, purposeful, and prosperous fulfilling life. You see our path is not set in stone, we are infinite beings, light-beings, souls who have chosen to incarnate and be here on earth at this precise time. What future can we now create personally, collectively, and for our beautiful planet?

May the light of your soul and the wisdom of your heart guide you always to greater love, and joy as you remember more of the magic of who you truly be and follow your bliss.

Much love from my heart to yours

Kimberley

PS: Thanks for reading! If you enjoyed this book or have found it useful, I'd be very grateful if you'd post a short review on Amazon, which will help others to find this book. Your support really does make a difference and I read all the reviews personally and these will support me to create even better future content. Thanks again for your support and look out for my next book in this Soul Journeys series, which will be out soon, where I will be sharing more Galactic Adventures.

PPS: If you'd like further support on your Soul's Journey or embracing and embodying your full potential and creating the life and business of your dreams, please do check out the resources page at the back of this book and connect with me on my social media channels, Facebook groups or via my website for further resources.

Book Meditation Bonuses: https://bit.ly/SJ1BookBonus

www.KimberleyLovell.co.uk

Lakota Prayer

My Native American name, given to me by my Native American spirit guide, Redwing, and other Lakota Sioux Chiefs, is Rainbow Weaver.

Wakan Tanka, Great Mystery
Teach me how to trust
My heart
my mind
my intuition
my inner knowing
The senses of my body
The blessings of my spirit
Teach me to trust these things
So that I may enter my Sacred Space
And love beyond my fear
And thus, Walk in Balance
With the passing of each glorious Sun

Mitakuye Oyasin – To All Our Relations

According to the native people, the sacred space is the space between exhalation and inhalation.

To walk in balance is to have heaven (spirituality) and earth (physicality) in harmony.

Resources

Soul Journeys Book 2: Galactic Adventures will be launching soon. Stay tuned!

Author's Website: www.KimberleyLovell.co.uk

Soul alignment/energy healing, hypnosis, business coaching/mentoring training programmes

Quantum Hypnotherapy Training
https://www.kimberleylovell.co.uk/training/quantum-hypnotherapy-training/

Book a quantum hypnotherapy soul journey or quantum leap hypnosis session here

https://www.kimberleylovell.co.uk/quantum-hypnotherapy/

Soul Journeys Ascension Healing Programme
https://www.kimberleylovell.co.uk/ascension-healing-programme/

Soul Journey Group Sessions
https://www.kimberleylovell.co.uk/soul-journey-group-sessions/

Facebook: https://www.facebook.com/kimberley.lovell

YouTube: www.youtube.com/user/KimberleyLovell

Past Life Regression Videos Playlist

https://youtube.com/playlist?list=PLvb3_ANaCvoGUWhc
mPEXQhPFoMjbgeLPM

Soundcloud https://soundcloud.com/kimberley-lovell-1

https://soundcloud.com/kimberley-lovell-1/tracks

About the Author

Kimberley is a spiritual intuitive, multi-dimensional channel, life coach, and business mentor with a background in psychotherapy, hypnotherapy, healing, coaching and teaching. She has worked with thousands of clients and students worldwide.

Kimberley lives in Bournemouth, Dorset, in the UK, with her partner, and her beloved Birman cat. She is a keen nature and wildlife photographer and can often be found in the forest with wild horses, ponies, donkeys, her crystals, and the trees.

Visit her website. https://www.kimberleylovell.co.uk/

Printed in Great Britain
by Amazon

78459354R00139